Praise for *Yoga for the Creative Soul*

"I'm dazzled. *Yoga for the Creative Soul* is more than a program or philosophy. It's a gift, merging the tenets of ancient and yoga-based psychology with the expressive arts and personal healing… In this blessed book, Erin presents us with an all-inclusive path to joy."
—Cyndi Dale, author of *Llewellyn's Complete Book of Chakras*

"A DIY guide full of exceptional exercises to awaken your best and most creative self… *Yoga for the Creative Soul* will help you to gently release fear, embrace change, gather courage, and overcome your inner perfectionist."
—Amy B. Scher, author of *How to Heal Yourself When No One Else Can*

"Erin Byron expertly guides you through fun-filled, creative workouts that are not only enjoyable but transformative. Encouraged by one of the exercises, I found myself happily skipping down the street, something I haven't done in a very long time."
—Sherrie Dillard, author of *Sacred Signs and Symbols*

"*Yoga for the Creative Soul* is a must-read for artists of life! Each one of us is looking to live to our fullest potential and this book is a practical guide on that path."
—Robert Butera, PhD, author of *Yoga Therapy for Stress and Anxiety*

"In *Yoga for the Creative Soul*, Erin Byron unlocks the key to the creative essence which is within each and every one of us, regardless of what external form it takes. This book is a guide to the process of finding that creativity and keeping it flowing."
—Servet Hasan, author of *Life in Transition: An Intuitive Guide to New Beginnings*

"In her new book, *Yoga for the Creative Soul*, author Erin Byron uses her extensive knowledge of yoga, the expressive arts, and psychotherapy to help her readers develop or release their natural creativity. This is a refreshing look at the emotional possibilities yoga can open."
—Jeanne Van Bronkhorst, author of *Dreams at the Threshold*

"I am impressed with how this book provides such an immediate and practical guide to accessing our wellspring of creativity. Everyone can benefit from this accessible map to exploration and expression."
—Gary Diggins, author of *Tuning the Eardrums: Listening as a Mindful Practice*

"*Yoga for the Creative Soul* is a call to delight in the transformative and liberating power of yoga by laying down the self-conscious fear-based ego and picking up the valuable art of play-driven vulnerability and authenticity, the balance between action and acceptance that can enable us to truly find and live our creative dharma, our life purpose."
—Dr. Ginger Garner, founder of the Professional Yoga Therapy Institute and author of *Medical Therapeutic Yoga*

"I love books that give you practical tools for transformation. And this book is full of them! In it, you'll find ways to heal yourself, inspire your creativity, and manifest your desires—all while unifying mind, body, and spirit!"
—Tess Whitehurst, author of *The Good Energy Book*

"*Yoga for the Creative Soul* is an inspirational wake-up call for the animating principle that we all long to express. Erin Byron shares ancient yogic concepts in a way that is both simple and profound, and offers clear insights that will illuminate the creative path for all ages and levels."
—Kristen Butera, RYT500, C-IAYT, author of *Yoga Therapy*

"This book is a gem for waking up your creative self using the principles and practice of yoga therapy. Accessible, inspiring, and fun, it is a unique resource for artists, entrepreneurs and anyone who wants to live a full, unabashed life."
—Rachel Krentzman, PT, C-IAYT, author of *Yoga for a Happy Back*

"Is your body longing for more meaningful expression? Erin Byron gives you lovely, creative ways to discover your body and yourself more deeply."
—Deborah Sandella, PhD, RN, author of *Goodbye Hurt & Pain*

"Erin Byron offers a unique and much-needed tool to awaken and ignite the creative fire. Heartfelt, imaginative, and highly accessible in its writing, this book is a must-have for everyone looking to dream and live in vivid color."
—Melanie Klein, co-editor of *Yoga and Body Image*

YOGA

for the

Creative Soul

About the Author

Erin Byron, MA, is a psychotherapist, enlightenment activist, and engaging speaker who has studied yoga psychology and expressive arts for twenty years. She is one of the founders of Comprehensive Yoga Therapist Training, specializing in mental health and clinical skills, and author of numerous books and articles on yoga, meditation, and resiliency. Erin brings laughter, creativity, and play into all of her writing and lectures as she connects you to the joy of what is possible in life. www.ErinByron.com

Other Books with Erin Byron

Yoga Therapy: Theory and Practice (Routledge)

Yoga Therapy for Stress and Anxiety

Llewellyn's Complete Book of Mindful Living

Yoga Therapy for Arthritis (Singing Dragon)

To Write to the Author

If you wish to contact the author or would like more information about this book, please write to the author in care of Llewellyn Worldwide, and we will forward your request. Both the author and publisher appreciate hearing from you and learning of your enjoyment of this book and how it has helped you. Llewellyn Worldwide cannot guarantee that every letter written to the author can be answered, but all will be forwarded. Please write to:

Erin Byron
℅ Llewellyn Worldwide
2143 Wooddale Drive
Woodbury, MN 55125-2989

Please enclose a self-addressed stamped envelope for reply,
or $1.00 to cover costs. If outside the USA, enclose
an international postal reply coupon.

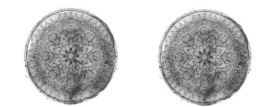

YOGA

for the

Creative Soul

*Exploring the Five Paths of Yoga
to Reclaim Your Expressive Spirit*

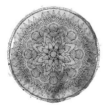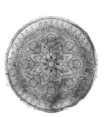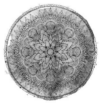

ERIN BYRON, MA

Llewellyn Worldwide
Woodbury, Minnesota

FIRST EDITION
First Printing, 2018

Book design by Bob Gaul
Cover design by Howie Severson/Fortuitous Publishing

Llewellyn Publications is a registered trademark of Llewellyn Worldwide Ltd.

Library of Congress Cataloging-in-Publication Data
Names: Byron, Erin, author.
Title: Yoga for the creative soul: exploring the five paths of yoga to
    reclaim your expressive spirit / Erin Byron.
Description: First Edition. | Woodbury: Llewellyn Worldwide, Ltd., 2017. |
    Includes bibliographical references.
Identifiers: LCCN 2017034514 (print) | LCCN 2017044357 (ebook) | ISBN
    9780738753713 (ebook) | ISBN 9780738752181 (alk. paper)
Subjects: LCSH: Yoga. | Yoga—Psychological aspects.
Classification: LCC RA781.67 (ebook) | LCC RA781.67 .B97 2017 (print) | DDC
    613.7/046—dc23
LC record available at https://lccn.loc.gov/2017034514

Llewellyn Publications
A Division of Llewellyn Worldwide Ltd.
2143 Wooddale Drive
Woodbury, MN 55125-2989
www.llewellyn.com

Printed in the United States of America

Disclaimer

THIS BOOK CONTAINS INFORMATION that is intended to help the readers be better-informed yoga practitioners. It is presented as general advice. This book is not intended to be a substitute for the advice of a physician or a psychologist/psychiatrist. Before beginning any new exercise program, it is recommended that you seek medical advice from your healthcare provider. The reader should consult with his or her respective provider in any matters relating to physical or mental health. The information in this book is meant to supplement, not replace, proper yoga *asana* training. Like any physical activity, yoga can pose some risk of physical injury if done improperly. The author and publisher advise readers that they have full responsibility for their safety and should know their limits. Before practicing *asana* poses as described in this book, be sure that you are well informed of proper practice and do not take risks beyond your experience and comfort levels. The publisher and the author assume no liability for any injuries caused to the reader that may result from the reader's use of the content contained herein and recommend common sense when contemplating the practices described in the work.

Acknowledgments

I AM SO THANKFUL to the countless people who contributed to shaping my life and learning. Each moment passed has brought me to this one and I am appreciative.

My mom, Donna, has been instrumental in supporting my journey as a psychotherapist, yoga studio owner, artist, homemaker, and healthy, friendly person. Thank you, Mom, for leading by example and for your tireless generosity, humor, and love. My dad, Don, for imparting values of hard work, education, and service. You taught me a lot about being an effective leader. My little brother, Kyle Byron, for being a superlative coach, cheerleader, and teammate. You inspire me every day to eat healthy, stay strong, care, and make a joke. To my cottage family for nourishing my child self then and now.

Robert (Bob) Butera. I say it all the time … because it is so: No Bob—no Erin. If the phrase "He taught me everything I know" can be true, it applies here. Thank you, Bobji, mentor, colleague, and friend. To Gita and Gail Laidler for introducing us and to the Yoga Institute of Mumbai for authentic teachings in tradition, self-reliance, and the ease of a pure practice—and for your role in sculpting Bob the yogi.

To the authoritative shaman and sweet smoochy, Peter Arcari, there is no end to my thankfulness. Because of you, I understand love. I get to talk esoterics, art, magic, and the meaning of all things every day … plus sunflowers! You are patient, wise, and a riot. Thank you for a home of creativity and wisdom.

To Joshua and Nathan Arcari, two of the best people I know. It is an inspiration to watch you trust yourselves and follow your artistry. Joshua, your precise forethought, unique eye, and layers of brilliance remind me to be brave, keen, and prudent. Nathan, you amaze me with your ability to read the moment and simply state its highest truth (and similarly give every one of your sculptures a soul). Each of you is a gift … wrapped in a present … wrapped in a gift.

To Kristen Butera, who teaches me what I am made of. Thank you for loving all parts of me—even the ones you haven't met yet. This balance of love, laughter, hard work, theorizing, applying, cooking, dancing, scheming, walking, moon-gazing, wave-riding, chalk-smearing, debating, unwinding, gif-ing, learning, lazing, cocreating, and communing serves me well!

To the many teachers who dedicated their lives to understanding through daily practice, thank you for sharing your true discoveries. To R. Duff Doel, Stephanie Scheid, Ria Caro, Andy Handley, and Ollie for insight into *pranamaya kosha* and the ways I may perceive and heal on that energetic level. To author and musician Gary Diggins for exemplifying life as an artist and enlightenment activist. To the team at Haliburton School of Art and Design for the weeks of inspiration, notably Julie McIntyre and Markus Alexander.

To Amy Reusch and Erin Strike for sharing creative space. To Sam Turton for curiosity and keen perspectives. To Ryan Doel, M. OMSc., for health support and education. To Jalen Seguin for being a mirror and dancing rock; to James Perly for strength; to Richard Willis for the heart of possibility.

To the team at Llewellyn Publications, especially the lovely, creative Angela Wix and patient, hawk-eyed Stephanie Finne.

Thank you to my Yoga Therapy colleagues and students, the International Association of Yoga Therapists, and the team of Comprehensive Yoga Therapy, for creating a vision and value for yoga in society. Staffan Elgelid, Libby Piper, Erika Tenenbaum, Shelly "The Connector" Prosko, Helene Couvrette, Steffany Moonaz, Marlysa Sullivan, Alison Braithwaite, Linda Boryski, Sarah Garden, Kristie Norquay, Marj Haire, Brittanya Beddington, Susan Tranmer, Jan Debenham and Shauna Ellerby, Tiffany Barrett Eyamie, Cassi Kit, Ginger Garner, Matt Taylor, Jen Collins Taylor, Michelle Peddle, John Kepner, and many others—you know who you are.

To those who kept things afloat during the transition: Gena Marta, Karen Van Eyk, Ronna Yallup, Erin Parkin, Mary Keefe, Jeff Lyons, Nora, Karen Camara, Debbie Grimm, and all the teachers and students who practiced karma yoga and purified their hearts, minds, or lives through participation. Thank you!

To the many students who reinforced and elaborated everything I know about yoga. You teach me innumerable perspectives and applications of our tradition. Thank you for your curiosity, methodology, and dedication. I am especially grateful to those of you who have stayed close throughout the years. Each student is dear to me and it is warming to remain a part of your life.

Thank you all for supporting me and the creation of this work.

Contents

Exercise List

Introduction

Yoga Therapy for the Creative Soul

Do you dream in color?

As a creative person, it might be unfathomable to you that some people dream in black and white or don't care what shade they paint their bathroom or refrain from singing and dancing when they clean the kitchen. As it turns out, not everyone is in touch with their creative essence.

How do you know if *you* are a creative person? There is a simple test for this: Do you exist? If the answer is anything other than no, then you are creative.

The operating premise is that we were created; thus, we are of Creation (however you define that word). Since we are of Creation, each of us is connected to a powerful creative force greater than ourselves.

Despite this truth, it's natural for a creative person to go through dry spells. Even you may have gone through phases where you can't settle on what song to listen to, aren't sure what to draw, or are no longer interested in the color of autumn's changing leaves. The reality of being a creative person is that most of us possess only a tenuous connection to inspiration. True, flowing brilliance can be fleeting. However, it doesn't have to be.

Rather than an elusive force, inspiration can be a sustained flow, like hydropower. When we are in touch with our creative essence, we are able to draw from the power grid. Whether you are someone who has never written a line, danced a step, or drawn a picture, or you are a professional artist who needs a steady stream of ideas, this book can support you in following a personalized approach to tapping into your own creative wellspring. You don't even have to be experienced in self-expression, art, or yoga—this book is written for the average person. Although, in the case of creative people, there is no "average"! This book is for all readers, no matter your age, beliefs, creative abilities, or physical fitness. Effective yoga philosophy and practices combine with expressive arts and personal reflection to guide you through a process of self-discovery and creative freedom.

Origins of *Yoga for the Creative Soul*

When I began my Master of Arts studies, my focus was to relate trauma healing to expressive arts. I had recently discovered the power visual expression has in releasing information and emotion that is held behind heavy walls. It was inspiring to see colors and shapes so clearly express what I barely had a verbal sense of. Words had always been my fortress. Since I began composing fables at eight years old, I knew I wanted to be a writer. Yet my journaling sessions often failed me as I endeavored to express my deeper pain or understand where it came from. Images set me free and told the tale.

Despite this power, I found within a year of grad school that my true inspiration was where I had worked for years: with the body. At the time, I had been attending bioenergetics therapy for four or five years and enjoying yoga for two. These body-mind approaches were helping me not only move stored trauma out of my cells but also fill them back up with health, relaxation, and care. Ultimately, my Master of Arts thesis was "Yoga Therapy for Post-Traumatic Stress" and this launched me into an enjoyable career as a psychotherapist, yoga teacher, and, eventually, studio owner. While I continue to train and mentor yoga teachers, meditation teachers, and Comprehensive Yoga Therapists, it is in balance with a creative life where I write in the genres of fiction and yoga therapy. I turn to my visual creations for investigation, solace, and inspiration, and I have spent the last few years leveraging that combination to build the life of my dreams.

I believe that each of us, when we truly listen to ourselves and act accordingly, can create the life of our dreams. I do not believe this is done in selfishness. When we investigate and heal our pain (or "burn our karma"), there is a flow of enlightened joy, gratitude, and compassion that comes into us. We interact with other humans and the planet itself with more reverence and appreciation; everyone, including us, benefits from this. When we understand the joy that is possible and see suffering in the world, we are less likely to tolerate it.

Artists have always been the conscience of a culture and a culture well-measured by how it treats its artists. As you connect to your own creative essence, your everyday life is likely to become evermore harmonious with your inner visions and the world around you. This means you are affecting change simply by the uplifted presence you carry. I think of this as Enlightenment Activism—the self-realized person acts to bring improvement to the world (be it in their own being, home, work environment, or local/global society). The inspiration of Enlightenment Activism is what brought this book into being.

This yoga therapy book is based on yoga teachings and techniques that have been recommended for generations. Although society has changed, these ancient approaches to well-being remain potent and effective. The expressive arts components draw on the creative essence that is in all of us.

The Creative Process

Think of creativity like a river. When there is no dam, the water flows unimpeded—fresh, bubbly, and musical. This is like us when our own creative juices are flowing; we feel powerful, beautiful, and like we can go anywhere with our ideas. All is possible! When the creative flow is dammed, however, we feel as stuck as that barricaded force of water—trapped and unmoving. Let us keep in mind that dams exist for a reason. Whether it is to house beavers so they can procreate or harness water for hydropower, even dammed rivers are still in some kind of creative process.

The same is true of ourselves. When we feel like the river of creativity has dried up or the waters are caught behind a dam, understand that this is merely a diversion. Even though it's not flowing the way we wish it to, the creative process is still in action. The juices have been harnessed and when we work with, rather than fight against, all aspects of the creative process, we connect with greater depth and acceptance to our own true creative essence. The expressive arts and yoga therapy exercises of this book will give you practical tools to do just that.

Comprehensive Yoga Therapy not only pinpoints areas of imbalance but also applies yoga philosophy and techniques to create sustained and progressive improvement in all areas of your life. Throughout this book I offer exercises to help rebalance your life for the purpose of activating your authentic creative voice—there is even a quiz relating your basic biological urges to your lifestyle choices. These exercises are designed to help you see your life from new perspectives, shift your thinking, and understand what powerful action steps you can take to begin improving your life immediately. You don't have to do all of the exercises in the book; however, to read the book and not do any exercises could be likened to prepping a delicious meal and not cooking it.

What Is Comprehensive Yoga Therapy?

Comprehensive Yoga Therapy is a specific kind of yoga therapy. The yoga therapy field is recognized as a scientifically valid approach to physical and mental health. Comprehensive Yoga Therapy is derived from Classical yoga and is accessible to all people, no matter their age, weight, or abilities. Comprehensive Yoga Therapy seeks to identify areas of imbalance in your life and help you practice the kind of self-reflection that motivates true, lasting change. Based on the timeless principles of Classical yoga, Comprehensive Yoga Therapy has a wealth of tools to support you in restoring balance. Yoga postures are one part, as are breathing, relaxation, and philosophy. The real power comes from harnessing the mind/feelings, intellect, and creative personal resources to effect change on a deeper level. Many of the practices in this book tap into the roots of your inspired self to connect to your creative essence, deep within your consciousness.

Comprehensive Yoga Therapy applies the self-realization practices of yoga to daily life and, in this case, creative living. Ancient healing methods are based on creating balance. Nowadays we do a yoga class alongside other people, but a personalized yoga plan for well-being has to be unique and incorporate not just postures but breathing exercises, relaxation, and, most importantly, the power of the mind. That's what this book provides!

The majority of people in modern society are healthy, but disconnection from our creative essence can slowly lead to health imbalances. Comprehensive Yoga Therapy offers a structure for preventative health care in the "Three Ps": Proactive, Participatory, and Personalized.

The 3 Ps of Comprehensive Yoga Therapy	
Proactive	Be empowered to take control of the lifestyle factors that predispose you to physical/mental/emotional/spiritual ailments
Participatory	Be engaged in and personally responsible for effecting positive change in all areas of your life
Personalized	Be viewed as an individual and receive uniquely meaningful tools to support your physical, energetic, mental, intellectual, and spiritual health

Whether you are new to yoga or an adept, this book is designed for you. Practice the yoga postures in a comfortable way, so you enjoy using your body and there is never pain. Sometimes the poses don't give you detailed specifics. This is intentional. More often than not, it doesn't matter if your arms lower to the sides or the front, for example, or if you inhale or exhale to get yourself into a movement. What is most important is your awareness of sensations and messages from your body as you move. It was awareness that brought *asanas* to the ancient yogis in the first place.

If you are familiar with yoga postures, you may notice that some of the names do not match the ones you are familiar with from class. Also, modern yoga postures may not have Sanskrit names. Different styles of yoga have different names for the same posture or the same names for different postures. After developing a tradition for thousands of years, you can imagine how some discrepancies may arise; hold them lightly and set your mind to your own inner process.

You do not need a yoga therapist to work through this book, which was written for the average reader to gain great benefit. That said, this book is not meant to replace professional medical or psychological advice. Continue working with your care providers and seek other help as it would benefit you. If you have any physical or mental health issues, please consult professionals. Should you wish to connect with a yoga therapist, check out the recommended resources at the end of this book for information on finding your own Comprehensive Yoga Therapist.

How to Use This Book

Start anywhere! *Yoga for the Creative Soul* guides you through a transformative process. Although this book was written in a linear, systematic way, you can jump around it however you want—read it in random segments, back to front, or by matching page numbers to your favorite numbers. Your journey through this book is directed by your own intention, created in chapter 1, Motivation & Movement. Through part

1's perspectives and practices, you will remove the obstacles that inhibit your creativity by exploring and weeding out their deeper roots. With fewer hindrances, part 2 assists you in discovering and tending creative parts of yourself and part 3 integrates it all into a joyful, thriving life.

Yoga's ancient philosophies and techniques appear here in a way that is relevant for the modern world. Go to the chapters and pages that are most relevant to your current questions and struggles. If you already feel strong in an area that we are discussing, skip it and go to the content and exercises that address your personal areas of need. You can always come back and read over the places you missed as your self-understanding deepens and you crave more information. If an exercise in the book seems too complex, boring, or irrelevant, leave it and attend to the ones you are ready to work with or value. Not all aspects are useful to all people and I considered as much variety as possible while writing this book. You may discover that some parts are targeting exactly what you need and are going through right now, while others may be relevant at other times in your life. You are welcome to personalize your journey through this book.

You will likely focus on chapters that relate to your disposition. For example, the work-oriented may follow chapter 6, Via Purpose; the emotional, chapter 8, From the Heart; one struggling with addiction may resonate with chapter 4, Toward & Away; and an alchemist could focus on chapter 14, Being. Different people operate through different filters and this can change through the course of life. Those who focus on chapter 12, Play Is a Need, for example, likely filter life through the body. While those relating to chapter 13, Human, approach life through the psyche. Follow your own frame of reference while also considering points of view and tactics from the other paths as they ignite your creative force.

It is best to get a journal of some kind for working through this book. You can have fun with this and select a notebook or sketchbook with an inspiring cover. Perhaps you can paint or collage your own cover on top of a generic blank book. You may get a special colored pen set to make writing or drawing in the journal more enticing. You can use this activity journal not only for completing the exercises of this book but also for your own creations, rants, visions, questions, affirmations, thoughts, and intentions.

The book is designed with a wealth of exercises so you can choose the ones that are most beneficial to your personal journey at any given time. When you complete the exercises, be honest about how your life is now, not how you want it to be or how it used to be. This gives you a realistic starting point and helps clarify the next steps to unleashing your creativity. Be willing to admit that some aspects of your beliefs contribute to creative stagnation and be willing to make a creative life. I suggest that you revisit this book time and again throughout your life—as you deepen and change, so will the benefits you receive from the exercises.

You will gain new insights about yourself, spirituality, and creative essence. Throughout this book, you have the chance to use many different tools that yoga tradition offers. In part 1, we address the blocks to creativity. Yoga psychology calls these hindrances *klesas* and lists five of them. The *klesas,* or obstacles, are ignorance, egoism, attachment, aversion, and fear. Once we stoke your motivation in chapter 1, the rest of part 1 gives you opportunities to explore what dampens that fiery enthusiasm and how to apply creative and yogic strategies to lessen its impact. In part 2, you have multitudinous opportunities to connect with hidden aspects of yourself. These forgotten or concealed pieces often hold a powerful current of creative juice. We investigate where each of the Five Paths of Yoga leads us as we traverse the inner landscape. Part 3 of this book guides you through practical, personalized ways of using creativity to create the life of your dreams, every day. When connected to our creative force, each of us has great opportunity to impact our own lives, the lives of our loved ones, and the world at large. Through interactions with all five layers of your being (the yogic concept of *koshas*), this book supports you in calling your dreams into reality.

Each chapter includes elements of yoga psychology, expressive arts (including but not limited to drawing, writing, dancing, humming, cooking, and finger painting), breathing, postures, meditation, relaxation, and self-inquiry. Usually, we give you a range of options for how to express or investigate; you are encouraged to experiment and trust your interest and enthusiasm.

At the beginning of the book there is an exercise list for each chapter, so you can quickly find techniques that work for you. Yoga posture practices are clearly indicated in this list. It also helps you revisit the book over time, reiterating what was important to you but may have slipped away, and giving you the chance to re-engage with practices that stir your creative essence. Much is to be gained from the creative explorations and modern-day applications of this book. Conversely, if you wish to know about the principles and find your own ways of connecting from there, it is all right to think about the philosophy and skip the exercises or make up your own. Use what fits for you and apply the aspects that make sense and improve your life.

You will notice italicized words throughout the book. These words are from the tradition of yoga, in the ancient language of Sanskrit. There are no direct translations for these words; however, we have included a glossary to begin to define them for you. If you choose to deepen your study of yoga, broadening your understanding of these concepts may be important. For now, notice how these concepts support your creativity and happiness.

It's in your power to decide how you want your life to be. I wrote this book to put you in alignment with the truth of your life and who you are. I believe that when you are invested in creating the life of your dreams, you are a part of making the entire world better. May your insights from reading and reflecting on what follows bring much creative power and joy. You can create whatever you wish!

Part 1
The Path of Creativity

WE BEGIN *Yoga for the Creative Soul* with a journey through the obstacles that stand between us and our true, expressive Selves. You may not yet believe that you are an expressive or creative person. Trust that if you have picked up this book, it is a calling from that mysterious place within that impels all creative action.

The Path of Creativity is a mystifying one. No two paths are alike. In fact, the more unique your expressions and creative outputs, the more likely it is that you are in touch with your true inner creator. This requires courage, however. Especially in the beginning, reaching into the depths of yourself to pull out some form of "art" can feel like swimming against an unseen current. Let the idea of "art" go for right now. Anytime a voice in your head starts talking about art or related concepts such as aesthetics, balance, harmony, or any other external judgment, shift your focus to the *process* of creating something and expressing yourself.

For the purpose of this book, and for the sake of your creative soul, reset your focus to the ideas of *creativity* and *self-expression*. They are a more honest filter through which to view your output. The part of us all that paints, writes, cooks, dances, etc., has its own personalized preferences and approach. As soon as we apply a vision of technique or outcome to that one-of-a-kind self-expression, we begin to take creativity out of the process.

This book is more about the process and about learning to keep the creative flow happening. This begins with chapter 1, Motivation & Movement, and carries on by addressing the five main obstacles in yoga philosophy that stand between who we think we are and who we really are. These spiritual hindrances are addressed in chapters 2 to 5: Resistance & Clearing Ignorance; I, Me, Mine, Divine; Toward & Away; and, finally, the interference of Fear.

Read on, and enjoy part 1 as it supports you in removing the obstacles that stand between you and a connection to your creative zest for life. You can explore the beliefs, experiences, and proclivities that limit your free expression and apply creative practices to learn more about why these barriers interfere with your unique personal journey. You will notice that some obstacles possess more power than others. It is okay for you to experiment with different barriers to different degrees on different days. Sometimes you may wish to examine deep personal challenges and other times take a gentle path to getting more insight about what you already have a handle on. Revisit part 1 anytime you lose touch with your creative process as a means of removing what may be standing in your way. Be playful and accepting—there is no right or wrong way to create. This is your journey. Enjoy it!

Chapter 1
Motivation & Movement

WHETHER YOU FEEL CONNECTED to it or not, you are a creative being. *Yoga for the Creative Soul* is based on the idea that you were created; thus, you are "of Creation" and therefore possess creative power. What creative power? That is unique to you. It may be painting or writing or comedy. You may have the ability to make people laugh, soothe them, or help them feel motivated. Perhaps your creative power lies in how you use numbers, juxtapose colors, or cook. This chapter investigates and amplifies your motivation to express this creative Self—dormant or thriving—that is an aspect of your essential makeup. It is also designed to support you during the times you feel uninspired. Do you want to be more creative? Do you want to stay creative? Do you wish you could be creative again?

… Why *are you* reading this book, anyway?

Before we go any further, let's get that question answered. It is about to become important.

Exercise: Rapid Intention-Setting

Answer the following question in your journal without thinking much about it. Your mind may have already brewed some form of answer. We will continue to work with developing your intention; for now, just write down the first thing that comes to mind as you complete the following sentence (no one else has to know what it is!):

I am reading this book for the purpose of…

Good job! That may not be the full, clear, final answer but it is a valuable start.

You are reading this book for *you*. You are the only one who truly holds the insight, power, and resources to change your life and become more of the person you genuinely are! You have nothing to prove to anyone, so you are safe to record whatever thoughts and beliefs arise from deep within you. No one else has to know but it is important that you know your own mind. Self-knowledge and self-reliance are key concepts in yoga therapy.

Intention-Setting Part I: The Subtleties of Creation

In the exercise above, you identified a personal reason for reading this book. Intention is an important aspect of all yoga practice. *Samkalpa*, the Sanskrit word for intention, means to bring into being through focus and will. In other words, "make it happen." Like most Sanskrit words, however, *samkalpa* also has more subtle meanings and lifestyle implications than the English language can convey.

The prefix *sam* means "with, together, wholly" and calls to mind a sense of unity and completeness, just as we are complete when united with our essential, creative Self. *Kalpa* is sometimes defined as "the true path" or, from *klrip*, "to frame, invent, imagine, or compose." In other words, what we make up or create is tied to our own true path. We can understand *samkalpa* as a way of being with ourselves and unifying with a path of wholeness. The second, more subtle meaning calls upon the power of imagination: we frame a dream then invent its reality by way of our decisive action. Anything you've ever made or done started with an idea that you worked to complete. Intention helps us compose our lives purposefully as it focuses the power of our action. Within that creative act lives the assumption that any endeavor will be guided by our own truth. The following exercise supports you in honing a subtle intention.

Exercise: Expressing a Subtle Intention

The following questions poke at the idea of *samkalpa*. You may complete each sentence in a brief, written fashion or use each of them as a choreographic theme, title of a sketch, or journaling prompt. Express each of the following three queries with as much or as little detail as you wish.

This book could make me more whole by…

I know that being more creative, on my own terms, will improve my life by…

Something I often imagine for myself is…

Now that you have connected a deeper spiritual sense to what motivates your Path of Creativity, we will explore the true-to-life energies that make you want to be more creative.

Intention-Setting Part II: The Practicalities of Creation

When we attune to our true Selves—the needs and wants crying out from the soul—it becomes easy to create strong intentions. It is through this inception that we gain vigor and enthusiasm for the project: from the inspiration of an idea, through the courage required to begin, the care to come through the middle, the stamina to complete it, and the ease to put it to some good use (even if only for your own insight). There is a great deal of creative force in a strong intention. Truly knowing why we are doing something empowers and inspires our work.

Understand that *samkalpa*, as discussed in the previous section, not only gets us moving and focuses our energy on the chosen path but also helps determine outcomes. One with a creative soul may be excellent at perceiving potential outcomes. This could be why we creative types are often called "dreamers"; we see what is possible, believe in it, and take steps toward making it happen. With your intention, or *samkalpa*, the power of your imagination and the forces of wholeness ready themselves to support you on the journey through this book.

Exercise: Exploring Hopes & Possibility

When you chose this book, somewhere in your imagination hope sprang forth. Perhaps you imagined yourself back in the studio, painting prolific landscapes. Maybe you heard yourself singing again, even if only over a sudsy dishpan in the kitchen sink. You may have felt encouraged that you could fill in Act II of your novel or screenplay... Any number of hopes and visions may have arisen when you decided on this book for creative souls.

Step 1: Breathe deeply as you remember that moment. What magical treasures may arise from this process? What might you reclaim? Who could you become?

Step 2: Take another deep breath and amplify the sense of that initial spark. Imagine it filling your body, breath, and thought field as you connect to possibility. If you aligned with your creative Self, what wonderful things could happen in your life? Who could you be?

Step 3: Journal, draw, or dance this vision/sense of yourself. Be free and nonjudgmental. Let whatever wants to come out do so! Enjoy the flow of ideas. Trust the process and hopes that spring forth.

The Voices of Nay-Sayers

Did you notice anything fishy while you were performing the previous exercise? There may have been a suspicious commentary. A nay-sayer lives within you! We all have one...or several. I used to have a village of nay-sayers inside me. The little voices of nay-sayers—critical, mean, bullying, fearful, judgmental—have probably been with you for a long time. Nay-sayers will probably accompany you on your journey through this book; in fact, I hope they do. Those nay-sayers have a *lot* to learn about the creative process and there is no better time than now.

If you let nay-sayers dry up your spring of hope and you abandoned the previous exercise, please go back and give it another go. We'll wait right here for you...

Excellent. Welcome back. We're going to address nay-sayers more as the book continues. For now, treat those voices the way you do traffic noise or other voices in a crowded room—disregard them and focus on what is important to you. The nay-sayers' actual words are rarely important. For now, it is enough to distinguish those mean, scared, or hopeless voices from that of your authentic, creative Self; filter out the nay-sayers!

The voices of nay-sayers arise from a lifetime of programming. Through our family's, teachers', coaches', and supervisors' directive feedback, we learned to criticize ourselves. While these voices are useful when discerning whether our actions will cause harm or bring shame, they are *not useful* in our creative pursuits. When you express yourself from an authentic place, whatever comes out of you is perfect. I will give you experiential evidence of this as you continue through the book; for now, take my word for it. *The nay-sayers are not helping your creative soul.* Rather than expressing a frame for your inner truth, they probably arise from past external programming.

The Process of Change

Past programming affects us in numerous visible and invisible ways. Our everyday routines reflect our beliefs back to us. Some of these beliefs are self-created and others were implanted long ago. When we try to change, our deeply held beliefs and programming make themselves known. There are many obstacles to change and we will address these through the rest of part 1. As you read the following section, keep in mind a behavior or habit that interferes with your creative life. This could be spending too much time in front of the TV or computer, nursing an addiction, saying yes to things you don't want to do, or some other activity that takes your time but does not add much value to your life. First, understand that change itself is not a single action or shift; rather, change is a process.

The Transtheoretical Model (Prochaska & DiClemente 1983; Prochaska, DiClemente & Norcross 1992) is a scientifically proven paradigm that describes the stages we go through in the process of intentional change. Change, even when we want it, is challenging. It is normal to experience resistance or waning motivation. Typically, change occurs in measurable stages. This model applies to any kind of change we may wish for; the following section relates it to living a more creative life.

Pre-Contemplation Stage happens before you even think of a change. There is either a denial of the problem or an awareness of the problem with an unwillingness to change it. For example, you may be in the Pre-Contemplation Stage of something in your creative journey that will make itself known in a later chapter or exercise. Remain curious and nonjudgmental with yourself.

Contemplation Stage has broken through denial, so you are aware of the benefit of change, but it does not mean you are ready. You may be more aware of how your habit interferes with your creative life, and you spend time thinking about the problem, but you have mixed feelings about changing things. This is the time to weigh pros and cons of quitting or modifying behavior. It is normal for there to be some doubt about the long-term benefits associated with change, especially if there are short-term costs. It helps to remember that all things are changing anyway, and you create a better life for yourself when you choose and direct changes instead of being tossed about by random happenstance. The following exercise helps you engage with this phase of change.

 ### Exercise: Contemplation of Potential Change

Reflect on or journal out answers to the following questions. You may also choose to draw this as a comic strip or choreograph a routine that expresses the journey through this leg of the change process:

What do you hope to change as a result of reading this book?

You may check in with the intention you set earlier in this chapter and see how it relates.

What will you have to give up if you make that change?

What rewards may come from it?

Can you relate this change to your past programming? In other words, why do you have this habit in the first place? *Who taught you or where did you pick up the habit?*

What needs does it meet for you? Are there healthier or more inspiring ways to meet that need?

Why haven't you changed it already?

This exercise has set the stage for the next phase of change: *Preparation.* In the Preparation Stage, you have decided you need to change and are thinking about what, how, and when to do it. This is a planning phase where, despite fear and resistance, you are aware of the benefits of change and are figuring out how to make adjustments so that you can live more creatively. This is an important stage, as it offers you the opportunity to envision your life without the problem behavior and foresee obstacles and solutions before they arise.

Action is essential. This is the phase most people believe is change itself. Contemplating and preparing for a more creative life will not make a creative life: this only happens through action. In the Action Stage, you believe you have the ability to change and are self-reliant in the process. Your motivation is peaking. If you can complete this phase with kindness toward yourself and nonattachment to the results (try learning about yourself through the process instead!), the transition may be easier.

Maintenance is a phase of sustained action, where healthy change is practiced and continually reinforced until it becomes automatic and lasts for an extended period of time. You get good at avoiding temptations and moments of weakness and pursue creativity. Maintenance is most readily observed when you are immersed in a practice that serves you on all levels, as we establish throughout this book and focus on in part 3. By the time you are maintaining a changed behavior, you experience a "new normal" and likely perceive many profound benefits as a result of your efforts (even though you weren't attached to those results happening).

Maintenance is a nice place to be because you are aware of a deeper worth and creative meaning in daily life. By this phase, you are more patient with yourself. Even though you may still have thoughts of returning to your old behaviors, or minor slips, you recognize that it takes time to integrate change. Effort is still required in the Maintenance Stage, which leads to one of two places: *Relapse* or *Stable Behavior*. We will talk about those outcomes in a moment, but first, take some time to connect to who you will be when you are maintaining a creative life.

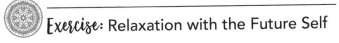

Exercise: Relaxation with the Future Self

As a creative person, you probably have many versions of yourself all playing out in the back of your mind. Sometimes it is hard to decide who we really want to be. Remember that anything is possible for you!

Step 1: Rest in a comfortable position and let the rise and fall of your breath soothe you.

Step 2: Imagine that you have completed this book and are truly connected to your creative soul. What kinds of things do you enjoy doing? How do you spend your free time? Who are your closest friends? Notice how it feels to be happy and a truer version of yourself. Enjoy the depth of your breath and physical ease as you witness your future Self: wise, creative, and free.

Step 3: Bask in this relaxation for as long as it serves you and return to it on a regular basis. You may envision maintaining the same future Self, strengthening that internal vision and external path, or you may explore many versions of your future Self, experimenting with a future that is yours to create.

When Maintenance fails, we *Relapse* into the recurrence of previous unhealthy behaviors. Relapse is a common aspect of change. Simply employ your strategies from the Action Stage or return to the Preparation Stage to explore how to firm up your process. There is much to be learned from Relapse when we approach it in this way. Usually, the process of returning to Maintenance will be faster as you have experienced a better life as a result of your changed behavior and are more motivated to cultivate creativity. The sooner Relapse is addressed, the more quickly it tends to be resolved.

Stable Behavior is apparent when the Maintenance Stage becomes automatic. This is the stage of Transcendence: life is better without the old habit and its return would seem foreign or not-self.

While the amount of time you will stay in each stage is variable, the tasks required to move to the next stage are not. Remember that "change" implies something happening over time. You may move through the phases in a nonlinear fashion, repeating or regressing as part of your process. See how change itself is a creative process.

Losing Steam

Similar to change, the creative process is also, well, a process! On the path of reclaiming your creative soul you may not always feel connected to inspiration. Sometimes it is beneficial to trust this disconnection as part of the process. Here in chapter 1, though, our focus is motivation! The rest of this chapter looks at ways you can reconnect to your creative essence.

When you are feeling dry, uninspired, or empty, it might relate to the Relapse Stage listed above. If we could tap into enthusiasm whenever we wanted, none of us would need this book, but that's not reality. Creativity, and changing ourselves back into the more creative people we are, involves a process. After all, it took us years to become the Internet-addicted, wine-swilling complainers that our happy, imaginative selves turned into. Sometimes we humans lose steam during this process. It can be difficult to keep the engine chugging and we don't always want to put in the effort. Even when we really want it, it is natural to fatigue on the way to our goal.

Two of the main reasons we lose steam, or relapse out of creativity, are (1) We are not clear about why we want the change in the first place, and (2) We don't want it enough. We will deal with number two in chapter 5, Fear. The following exercise addresses number one by helping you amplify your motivation by vitalizing your subtle energy and connecting your mind and body to your creative soul.

Exercise: Inspiring Breath: The Prolonged Inhale (*Puraka*)

Yoga therapy gives us many tools to adapt our state of mind and physiology. *Pranayama*, or breath/energy practices, are powerful because they link the mind and body and have an impact on our subtle energy. The following practice in known for increasing vitality, clarity, and enthusiasm. It is literally *inspiring*.

Note: Some people feel fatigued by this exercise. This is a sign that you are forcing the breath, rather than allowing the inhale to expand in its own way. If you feel tired or light-headed, stop the exercise immediately and breathe normally, lying down if necessary. You may choose not to attempt this if you are pregnant or have a vascular condition.

Step 1: Focus on the inspiration—by this I mean inhale. Every time your lungs fill, notice their movement and the associated movements throughout your body. Let the exhale take care of itself and continue noticing how your body breathes in. What happens in your abdomen, ribs, and chest? Can you feel something in your back? How about your pelvic floor or the base of your skull? As you continue to focus on the in-breath, what else do you notice in your body?

Step 2: Allow the inhale to elaborate. Feel it spread further and further through your body, carrying a sense of vitality and openness through your abdomen, chest, and back, right up to your head and out the extremities to the fingers and toes. Allow several breaths to distribute the inspiration through your body.

Step 3: Notice the thoughts and emotions that accompany this expansion. Trust the exhale to do its own thing and bring your mind back to the breath each time you inhale. You may choose to count the number of seconds of each inhale, adding a second each time the breath becomes comfortable at its current count. Do not force the breath or compete with yourself to make the inhales longer; relax into the process.

Step 4: On a fresh page, draw your inspiration as if it were an amusement park ride. What colors arose with this prolonged inhale? How did it move? What feelings did it give you? It's okay if your drawing is clumsy or doesn't come out on paper the way it looks in your mind (no thank you on the commentary, naysayers!). Enjoy the process of representing your influx of oxygen through color, form, and imagination!

Enthusiasm

We create not only through inspiration but through a pleasant sense of engagement and happiness. "Enthusiasm" is one of my favorite words because, for as much as it indicates a sense of joy and purpose, it literally means "the God within." Even in your darkest moments as an artist (whether your medium is acrylic paint, butter, or a vacuum: remember, you are an artist of life), there is a pleasure in the creative process. A sense of enthusiasm holds us connected to our creative soul through joy and purpose.

Joy is a theme you will see throughout this book. A person creating a true Self is inevitably going to connect with joy. The yogis remind us that the essence of each person is bliss (*ananda*). Creator—however you define that divine spark that put geometry in trees and made possible the platypus—also made us. We are of Creation and therefore creative by our nature. Yoga is a path of discovering your true nature. Creative expression is a path to the same discovery. By combining the modalities of yoga and creativity, this book gives you many opportunities for lightheartedness, art (expressive, not necessarily technique-based or skillful), and genuine connection to meaning. These features bring enthusiasm!

Parts of this book may challenge you or quell your enthusiasm as you clear out past pain and programming. Any time you feel disconnected from joy or your sense of purpose, remember the following exercise to reconnect and uplift yourself.

Exercise: Buoyancy: What to Do When You Get Weighed Down

I spent a lot of my childhood on different kinds of boats. We took enough trips around the Great Lakes that I was highly familiar with the idea of buoys. These flotation devices bobbed upon the blue-green water noting boat moorings, big rocks just below the surface, or, in the case of larger ones, where to locate the channel through the water and on which side to pass. Even our life jackets had "buoy" in the brand name. These bouncing markers helped keep us safe and above water.

We can all feel like we are being dragged under sometimes. In these times of overwhelm, despair, or apathy, it's beneficial to know which way is up. Any good seafarer who goes under knows to watch the bubbles. Those little capsules of buoyancy take a direct route to the top. By following the bubbles, we find our way to the surface and prevent ourselves from drowning. The following exercise helps you connect with a sense of buoyancy so you can keep yourself afloat in deep waters.

Step 1: Skip! If you don't know how to skip, try walking with an extra hop on each foot as your lifted leg swings gently forward. Keep your knees soft and land lightly on the balls of your feet. If skipping is not appropriate for your body, you can receive the same effects by standing in one place and lightly bouncing on the balls of your feet (quickly, lightly lifting and lowering the heels). In this option, the feet need never leave the ground.

If you are apprehensive about skipping through the super-market or while accompanying the children to school, do it after the sun has gone down and no one's around or from living room to kitchen and back or along the shoreline of a rolling ocean.

Step 2: As you skip (or bounce), notice the sensation in your breath and where you feel it most in your body. Acknowledge the rhythm of your heartbeat, steps, inhales, and exhales. Perceive the movement of energy within and around you, together with your thoughts and feelings.

Step 3: Find three words that describe what follows your skipping/bouncing practice. What colors are there? If it were the weather, what kind of day would it be? Hum the main "hook" or theme to the soundtrack of skipping.

Step 4: Skip s'more!

You have laid out a brief intention for the book, called upon an image of your future Self, explored the process of change, and experienced a practice to incite connection and enthusiasm. May your motivation be secure. Chapter 2 continues with the theme of connecting—or not—to the creative Self. Read on to explore what happens when we forget to tap into our own creative spirit and explore practical techniques to plug back in.

Chapter 2
Resistance & Clearing Ignorance

WHO ARE YOU, REALLY? If we wish to live a creative life, it is key to connect to the authentic Self. Our creative nature springs from an eternal truth within us: a center of hope, freedom, and unique expressivity. A parallel principle is at the heart of yoga: there is a true spiritual spark within each of us, whether we are aware of it or not. The ultimate role of a yoga therapist is to offer education and practices that promote self-realization and connect clients to that essential nature. The *Yoga Sutras* is one of the traditional texts of yoga. It is divided into four chapters, each containing numbered verses or "threads" (*sutras*). The *Yoga Sutras* teach that yoga is a process of uniting who we think we are with who we truly are. A simple way to think of it is this: when we align the "ego" (who we think we are) with the "true Self" (or soul, divine spark, inner creator—whatever makes sense to you) we are said to be in a state of yoga. Thus, harmonizing with our creative essence is a yogic path.

It's easy to move out of harmony with the true Self. Like a trombonist who stops listening to the unified sound of the orchestra, we fall flat and off-tempo when we do not connect with the various emotional chords, rhythms, and counterpoints in our own lives. Often this is not a conscious "checking out"; rather, it is something that happens over time through a series of habitual choices. Sometimes we create dissonance on purpose by resisting action.

In this chapter, we talk about the five main obstacles or hindrances that stand between us and our creative Selves and explore the impact of the first obstacle, as well as how to remove it. We get to know "resistance" a little better and examine how it is at play, either willfully or passively, in our own lives. Finally, we look at a fundamental piece of yoga philosophy, *karma*, and its role in obscuring our creative essence.

We have all known what was best and not done it, even when it was something we genuinely wanted to do! Sometimes this happens because of laziness or because we are excited about doing something else instead. There are times when resistance stems from a valid concern about moving forward—be truthful about whether you are avoiding something important or reluctant for a good reason. We might also resist because action is scary or our old mental programming and habits deter us. The last example, where we are operating from an automatic place, is identified as one of the main obstacles to connecting with our creative soul.

The Obstacles or Hindrances to Creative Connection

The *Yoga Sutras* teach that there are five main obstacles (*klesas*) that stand between us and our creative soul: ignorance (*avidya*), egoism (*asmita*), attachment (*raga*), aversion (*dvesha*), and fear of death (*abhinivesa*). These obstacles, or hindrances to our enlightenment, occur predictably in all people and appear in myriad forms. This chapter focuses on the primary obstacle, ignorance; the next three chapters cover the other four. Consider that any barrier to creativity stems from one of these *klesas*.

The primary hindrance, ignorance, does not speak to one's education. It is not a lack of information that stands between who we think we are and the true creative Self—it is the *ignorance* of the existence of the creative Self that hinders us. Although there is greater depth to the Vendanta philosophy than we shall cover here, you can think of it this way: if we are embodied souls and yoga is a path to identifying ourselves more with the soul and less with the body, then we must remember the existence of the soul itself. When the *klesa* of ignorance is at play, we have forgotten (or are ignorant of) the divine.

Exercise: Connecting with Your Spirit Self

Play this imagination game on days when, for whatever reason, you are feeling unwell. As you move through your day, completing boring, challenging, fun, or scary tasks, occasionally check in and ask yourself, "If I were a spirit, what would I do right now?"

Stepping outside of our usual frame of reference changes the entire picture. From the perspective of a spirit, you might perceive greater possibilities: "I would make up a song about listing this new inventory," "I would connect with my loved ones," "I would fly around the office dropping flower petals and honking like a goose… That would really make Janice laugh. Hahaha!"

From the perspective of a spirit, you may also notice things that human you doesn't pay attention to, like the paintings in an office hallway, how "wrong" a certain situation feels, or the beauty of a small tree outside your window.

Although the answer to "If I were a spirit, what would I do right now?" might be "Exactly what I AM doing," asking the question over time will alter the way you make big-picture decisions. All it takes to realize the creative soul is to remember to connect to the creative soul. Training ourselves to do that in everyday moments keeps us mindful, conscious, and creative the whole day through. Then, when it comes time, we shift our habits toward the creative being we truly are.

How can we connect with something we have forgotten even exists? If we get caught up in our stress, busyness, or day-to-day trials, our focus has shifted from the divine to the everyday. It does not take long before we are focusing more on bank accounts than sunsets, pop radio than composing. Finishing the grocery shopping becomes more important than cooking for an ailing neighbor. Our current society is set up to keep us focused on consumerism, which in turn distracts us from a quiet sense of true connection. Ergo, we grow ignorant of our own authentic, creative Self. Use the following exercise as one means of visioning a reconnection.

 Exercise: Uniting with Your Creative Essence

Many sages who have described their enlightenment experiences speak of it happening instantaneously…after years of dedicated practice, mind you. But when it happened, it happened all at once. For the purpose of this book, we are defining this state of enlightenment as union with your creative essence.

Step 1: Imagine yourself in an enlightened state—a sense of being in exactly the right place, of abundant well-being, of all things clicking perfectly together. Perhaps you have already had an experience like this or maybe you are calling on your imagination.

Step 2: Once you have an embodied sense of union with your creative soul, express it somehow. You may decide to play its melody, dance its sense, or sculpt its representation in clay. Choosing your preferred method of expression, form something that sheds a layer of ignorance and puts you in touch with your creative soul. Hold on to this sense of your enlightened self and allow it to encourage and inspire you in everyday life. Remember, your creative Self is already enlightened—waiting to be discovered within you! This connection is all that is required to remove the obstacle of ignorance.

The loss of connection, when ignorance is at play, is often accompanied by restlessness. The unfortunate nature of this is that our tendency is to seek solace outside of ourselves. We entrench ourselves even more deeply in the habits that cut us off from freedom and joy in the first place. Even if we recall the possibility of a spiritual, creative life, we resist the steps required to reconnect us.

Let's face it: we are excellent at self-sabotage. It might not always be intentional and it usually happens on a small scale; however, these little acts of interference, over a long period of time, lead to our despair. Imagine where you would be in life if you never procrastinated, indulged in substance use, or associated with people who bored you. It would be a different life. Don't get me wrong; I believe that there is a place for resistance and it serves some kind of self-protective purpose. However, resistance without awareness is spiritual ignorance. We have forgotten the true Self. The following yoga pose practice gives you the chance to align your creative Self with an embodied sense.

Exercise: Yoga Posture Practice: Anti-"Ignorance"

You may follow the *asana* sequence laid out below or create your own movement pattern. The key point of this exercise is to use the postures to knit your body and creative Self more closely together via your chosen intention/image.

Step 1: Look at the previous exercise, Uniting with Your Creative Essence, and find a word or image that represents the experience of connecting to your creative soul. Any symbol is fine, as long as it brings you greater spiritual or self-awareness.

Step 2: From a standing position, breathe in and fill yourself with that inspiring, aligned sense of creative connection. Use the word or image as a mind-focusing tool. Imagine that you are coming into alignment with the strong, open you-that-you-are.

Step 3: Palm Tree Pose (*Talasana*)—On the next inhale, raise the arms overhead and lift on to the balls of your feet (tippy-toes), as if you are reaching for that symbolic word or image way up high, using your entire body to grow taller. If it is safe to do so, you may hold your breath in as you stay in the uplifted, reaching posture. On an exhale, slowly lower the arms to the sides of your torso and lower your heels as you imagine carrying all that you require down from the heavens. Repeat this intentional action of lifting the arms and heels three to ten times.

Step 4: Standing Forward Bend (*Uttanasana*)—After the final exhale of the previous posture, place your palms together in front of your heart, as if to seal the symbol into your soul. (Note: The heart is a suggestion. You may benefit more from sealing them into your sacrum, root, throat, head, etc. Do what seems best for you.) As you hold your hands over this sacred place, begin to bow the head in reverence. Bend the knees as necessary as you allow the rest of the spine to curl forward more and more, forward bending toward the ground. Although your abdominals may brace your spine for safety, feel surrendered in this standing forward fold. Allow your resistances and doubts to let go as the back of the neck, torso, and legs relax. You may hold the breath out or breathe a few breaths as you hold the pose before inhaling to roll upward and open your arms to the sky. Instead, you may keep the posture dynamic: rising to standing with each inhale and releasing to a forward bend with each exhale.

Step 5: Plank/Half-Plank—If it suits you, place your palms on the floor while you are performing the previous, forward-folding posture. Step your feet behind you to a plank pose, so you are on hands and toes. If someone set a plank on your calves, it would touch you all the way along your back to the back of your head—a nice, long line. Lower your knees and hips to form an inclined plane, hands beneath the shoulders. Experience the ability in your arms and through the abdominal corset. Sense softness in your heart and the place between your shoulder blades, even as the back and chest are strong; this interplay of strength and softness help you balance the word or image in your body-mind system. You may have fun with various kinds of elbow bends, neck positions, or straightening the knees to return to full plank, keeping the subtle heart area open all the while.

Step 6: Bow Pose (*Dhanurasana*)—From your plank or half-plank position, bend the elbows to lower yourself all the way on to your abdomen, keeping your spine engaged all the while. Now you are lying belly-down on the mat. Do not force this next posture; enjoy the opening sense in front of your body and the strength in your back.

Bend the knees to bring the heels behind you toward your seat. Reach your arms behind you, as if you were going to hold your ankles (which you may decide to do). As you inhale, lift your knees off the mat, keeping them about hip-width apart and the toes toward the sky. Roll your shoulders and chest up, too. Imagine yourself poised like an elegant archer's bow: mobile in the open places and strong in structure. The muscles through the back of your body are engaged as your heart lifts forward and up and pelvis opens as the knees and feet rise. Take in an influx of energy from your word or image. Release by rolling the front of the spine back to the mat and setting the knees and feet down. You may flow in and out of this position on each breath cycle or hold for a few breaths before releasing, deepening your experience of a balanced, strong-and-soft connection to your creative Self.

Step 7: Seated Twist, legs extended—An optional transition from lying on your abdomen is to bend the knees and bring the hips back to the heels, keeping the chest and head on the mat as you rest in Child's Pose (*Balasana*). Roll the spine, torso, and head up to a perpendicular position with your legs—now you are seated.

Extend both legs in front of you, hip distance apart. Raise your arms to shoulder height in front of you, palms cupped and facing each other as if you were holding a beach ball. Keep the back tall and the legs long and strong as you gaze into the empty space between your open palms. Imagine filling that space with the qualities your word or image represents. Plainly perceive a shift in the energy or visual sense of what is in your hands.

Flex your toes toward the sky and press through the heels and thighs to strengthen your base. Holding your vision on the space between your hands, revolve to the right. Do your best to remain square on your sit bones and across the shoulders, keeping hands at shoulder height. Breathe deeply and look into the creative space your hands hold. Stay tall through the torso.

When you are ready, return to center and twist the other way. Stay aware of your breath and continue to focus your mind, gaze, and creative sense on the space between the hands. You may notice its presence continue to amplify. You can hold the twist, allowing yourself to continually explore and adjust for comfort, conditioning, and safety, or stay dynamic as you twist from side-to-side for a couple of minutes.

When you are through with this pose, you might imagine one of your hindrances in front of you. Set what you were holding symbolically between your palms next to that hindrance. Play with how your hindrance and intention interact. You may write a scene, dance, or do a puppet show about it when you are done with this sequence—or now works, too. Trust your inspiration—it's a beneficial habit in transforming resistance.

Step 8: Extended Side Bend—Stand up and bring your feet comfortably wide apart, arms to the sides at shoulder height. Engage the strength of your full body. As you hold power through the inside and outside of the arms and legs and the front and back of the torso, imagine imbuing that physical might with your image/intention. Body and intention are strong. Stay strong yet pliable as you side bend to the left. Arms may remain wide or you can bring the left hand down the side of your leg and the right arm alongside the ear. Open the right (top) side of your body and breathe even more of your intention into that space. Sense yourself becoming bigger and stronger, fully supported by the earth and enjoying the sense of reach. Repeat on the other side, bending right and lifting left, feeling at once open, mighty, and mobile. Remember to support the body with breath, perhaps breathing your intention as you open to it, reach for it, and hold it in your strength.

Step 9: Simply stand and feel how lovely it is to have a body, to move breath, to experience emotions, to create thoughts, and to be aware of a greater intentionality at play behind all those movements. Bask in this connection to your creative soul.

Staying Connected to the Creative Soul

Though the *Yoga Sutras* teach us that we are often ignorant to the existence of our true Selves, they do not tell us what to believe. Your direct experience of your creative soul, whatever it may be that enlightens you, is enough to plug you back into your true Self and wash away any resistance in the tide of inspiration.

From a yoga perspective, we are free from the *klesa* of ignorance when we remember that we are spiritual beings. Releasing ignorance about the existence of spiritual reality creates the possibility that there is a greater mystery at play than our puny five senses, selfish prejudices and desires, and fearful minds can fathom. Through the practice and guidance of yoga we shed our small personalities and unite with a larger, more truthful creative Self. It's easy to succumb to resistance if we are ignorant of the great mystery, our creative essence, and the possibilities it implies. Sometimes we act as if we do not want to connect to our creative essence.

Resistance can happen because we are not ready to align with the creative soul or live with some of the implications. Relationships will change, the budget might shift, free time activities look a lot different—ultimately, these alterations are a form of trimming the waste so you are left with the truth of who you are. Even though it is normal to resist changing and living in joy and creativity, once you have a visceral sense of why and how to do it, and how amazing it feels when you do, the resistance dissolves into that goodness. For example, the creative soul remembers that most things aren't worth stressing about; it can guide our choices and responses. In fact, creators consciously choose everything that's happening to them—either through action, nonaction, or mistake. We are actually the creator of this whole thing called life, but most of us are not consciously creating.

It's okay if you don't believe that last bit. Just imagine if it were possible: if you were a creative being (yourself a creation and your soul wishing to create and express), you could potentially create every minute of every day through your life choices. Even when things happen outside of your control you choose your perspectives and responses. What if you really were the creator in your life? What if, just maybe, things could turn out the way you want them to? The following practice continues to support your mindfulness around aligning with your creative soul.

**Exercise: Visualization, Music &
Movement for Creative Possibilities**

Just as we grow ignorant of our spiritual Self, so to do we forget the vast possibilities of our own lives. One of the many reasons it is frightening to change to a more creative life is that we have forgotten how much control we have over our decisions. It is normal for a sense of helplessness to overwhelm you as you begin to make creative changes and dream bigger dreams. You may wonder, *If it were possible for me to express myself and be more creative, why wouldn't I have done that already?* The biggest two barriers would-be creatives name are the dearest of resources: time and money. Let's play with what could happen if those material obstacles were removed. These steps help you dream a little bigger and a bit more surely.

Step 1: Answer the following question by listing as many things as you can in thirty seconds. You are welcome to repeat yourself; just keep writing as fast as you can for thirty seconds. Get set with pen and paper. Ready? *If anything were possible and there was nothing to fear, starting right now, what would I do differently?* [GO! Write down as much as you can without filtering yourself.]

Step 2: Put on one of your favorite, upbeat songs. From any standing position, read through the list, holding the corners of your mouth upward and showing your teeth. Let the feelings and images of these possibilities flow through you.

Step 3: Repeat your favorite song, or choose another, and perform an interpretive dance about the possibilities your mind has created. By processing your imaginings through body movement, you are helping to give them an active, joyful physical reality.

Continue to be curious about and believe in what is possible for you. I know it can be scary being responsible for our own lives. We will address personal responsibility in the next chapter. For now, let us continue to investigate why we resist our own sense of possibility and taking action on our dreams. What we believe about what is possible for us in life often stems from past programming. Each of us has our own ways of expressing or manifesting resistance. This often has to do with our predispositions, or *karma*.

The Role of Karma

Before getting into how your *karma* relates to resistance, let's clarify some misconceptions: First off, even though *karma* operates on the idea that "What goes around comes around," the wise do not seek "good *karma*." Furthermore, we apply spiritual intention and pure action to avoid "bad *karma*." Despite our best intentions, most karma is "mixed," or a combination of pain and pleasure, both of which could be returned to us in kind. Because we may already have what amounts to lifetimes of *karma* barreling down upon us, we don't need any more of it—not even the "good" kind.

Karma translates as "deed; action or former action that leads to results; or reaction, fruits," from the word *kri*, "to do." *Karma* is the act itself in addition to the outcome that arises from that act. Rather than seeking good, bad, or mixed *karma*, "*karma* neutral" is best, where we do not incur any more *karma* through our actions. (Some believe it is impossible for humans to be *karma* neutral, but we won't get into that here.) Our resistance patterns, be they procrastination, self-doubt, or some other form of sabotage, are a repeating *karma*. Like all *karmic* imprints, we can diminish the effects by understanding and accepting the underlying pattern. The following exercise helps you identify a portion of your creative resistance and express it.

Exercise: Identify & Express Creative Resistance

Through this process, you may release some *karma* as you move more in alignment with the truth of your whole, creative Self. It can be fun to revisit this exercise over the years as resistance or dry spells recur. You will continue to burn through layers of *karma*. Even though the core issue may remain the same, you will deepen your understanding of it—and by extension your creative Self—each time.

Step 1: Draw a circle the size of a piece of paper. Inside the circle, write down a project that is important to you that you aren't working on. This may be organizing the garage, learning how to grow rosemary, or touching up a watercolor painting—whatever you want to do but are not acting upon.

Step 2: Think of a time in your near or distant past when you did not complete a project that was important to you. This may have been something you were writing, sewing, painting … whatever. Write down that project. Repeat step 2 as many times as you can think of unfinished projects.

Step 3: As you read over those incomplete actions, notice what happens to your posture, breath, and thoughts. Exaggerate all three of these checkpoints, so that your thoughts become even more busy or self-deprecating. If your breath is quick, make it faster. If your posture is tense, tighten it even more. Exaggerate your reaction for as long as it takes to reach a peak (for example, your breath is as shallow as it can be, your body as small as you can wind it), between 20 and 120 seconds.

Step 4: Turn the paper where you recorded these unfinished tasks into a sculpture. Express via the paper what your mind, breath, and body were just expressing. Put all of that energy into the paper as you crumple, rip, fold, and play.

Step 5: Stand beside your sculpture. Imagine it is a representation of all the times you have looped around the same pattern. Allow the energy of those patterns to be sealed in that sculpture.

Step 6: On a fresh page, write down the very first time you remember resisting a task. This could be practicing how to tie your shoes, finding an item for show-and-tell, or writing a grade school report. Relax as you remember your young self knowing what needed to be done but not wanting to do it. Use your imagination to go deeply into that experience. It's okay if you take liberties with filling in the details. Since this is exclusively your journey (you won't accuse others of roles they may have played or need to prove what truly happened), you can use creative imagination to understand possibilities of what may have been happening within your young self. How did you feel? What did you believe, fear, or want?

Step 7: Use construction paper, tissue paper, or colored sheets in conjunction with the sheet where you wrote this memory to create another sculpture. Use your nondominant hand as much as possible to express what that child was going through.

Step 8: Return to your imagining of that first resistant experience, this time from a neutral point of view. Witness this child from the spiritual perspective of your creative Self, as we practiced earlier in the Connecting with Your Spirit Self exercise. See your child self in acceptance, compassion, and love as you watch the resistance play out. What about this situation or him/herself is this child ignorant of? What spiritual perspective soothes this situation? The answer may be a virtue, like courage or patience, or a spiritual need, like connection or support. Using the colored paper again, create a sculpture that represents the spiritual perspective soothing the resistance.

Step 9: Relate what you needed as a child to step 2, all those not-completed tasks, and what you need as an adult. Kinda similar, huh? That's an example of *karma*. Now you know, every time you resist, it is like another trip around the loop. Remember your child self and reach out to that version of your being in those moments when you "don't wanna." Sometimes resistance is valid—we need something else in the moment.

When we resist what is truly best, we are repeating *karma*. For whatever reason, some emotion or belief programmed into the back of our minds interferes with our will or ability to take action. Resistant behavior, which usually looks like some form of procrastination or running away, expresses an untruth in the moment and is based on an ingrained emotional experience or limiting belief. Instead, consider using truthful expression when resistance arises. Creative action of any kind is a tool to work through and resolve past issues—burn *karma*—and neutralize the impacts your past is having on your present life. The following exercise gives you a way to play with that.

Exercise: Breaking the Cycle of Resistance

If you are "getting in your own way" somehow, avoiding or fearing a creative task, see how things change after you do the following:

Step 1: Situate yourself as if you were going to complete the task you are resisting. If it's writing an essay, sit at your desk; if it's cooking supper, place yourself in the kitchen; if it's choosing on outfit for a big event, stand in front of your closet.

Step 2: Express your resistance however you want. Type out all of the reasons your essay is boring and doomed to fail. Sing a song to the veggies about preparing themselves. Dance and wave different outfits around the room or use them as puppets to explain why they may or may not be the best choice. Spend two to twenty minutes in any of these activities.

Step 3 (optional): Select a completely different modality and express how it felt to act out step 2. You may note what you learned or what made you curious. Acknowledge what did and did not ring true for you about the experience and what you heard yourself express. For example, "I have nothing to say for this essay" is more truthful than, "This is going to turn out terribly." Our resistance often arises from negative core beliefs and fears. Once you put them into the open, they start to lose their power. When we are aware of the *karma*, or the fears and habits associated with our resistant patterns, we have the power to change our future. "Future pain can be avoided," says the *Yoga Sutras*. This gives us hope that we can act to dissolve what *karmas* may be coming our way as a result of our past thoughts, actions, and reactions.

You may have noticed I recommended a great deal of playful expression in this chapter. One of the things that empowers resistance is a sense of seriousness, as if completing the project were the most important thing in the world. In truth, stakes are rarely that high. So you don't get through editing your film—there will be others. If you don't get your book to your publisher, the worst thing that happens is it doesn't get published. You will survive these things, and so will the people counting on you.

Are those your desired outcomes? I doubt it. Is it how you want to behave in the world? Probably not. Ultimately, however, the pressure is just a story. The true opportunity, the yogis teach us, is to know ourselves better through the struggle. Thus, even if the task winds up a failure, the process of learning and growing can be a victory.

Hopefully this chapter gave you more freedom to explore the pressure you put on yourself and how your resistance to working on your projects stems from forgetting that you are a creator—you have great possibility! As you face the *karma* that underlies your resistance and remove the obstacles to your true Self, you live evermore in alignment with creativity. You may notice that a thread of ignorance runs through all the other hindrances, too. In the following chapter, we will explore another of the five hindrances: egoism.

Chapter 3
I, Me, Mine, Divine

IN THE PREVIOUS CHAPTER, we explored the main obstacle that stands between us and enlightenment. It is forgetting there is such a thing as enlightenment! In other words, our perspectives, beliefs, and sense of connection dictate our experience of the divine in everyday life. The tradition of yoga does not carve a single path to enlightenment, nor does it specifically teach what divine presence is. For the purpose of this book, we are relating spirituality and the divine to the creative soul; ergo, the previous chapter helped open a deeper sense of meaning in and engagement with everyday life. Now that you are developing a pattern of connecting to spiritual purpose, we shall examine how your individuality fits into the great mystery of life. This chapter explores the *klesa* of egoism, describes an ancient philosophy of human makeup, and offers you experiences to unite your personality self with your creative soul.

When We, Ourselves, Are the Obstacle

According to the *Yoga Sutras,* the second hindrance, or obstacle, between you and your creative soul is "egoism" (*asmita*): confusing your body and mind for the divine mind. We all give too much power to our passing thoughts, at times, believing that story we weave is the entire truth of a situation. In reality, there are many perspectives outside of our own, including a vast divine perspective that may be beyond our human comprehension. A more obvious form of egoism is being too self-focused. In modern life, we often think of egoism as pomposity or arrogance, but in this case it simply means giving ourselves too much attention. The person who is preoccupied with self-loathing and despair is just as ego-centric as the insensitive narcissist. When our thoughts are caught up in ourselves—the "selves" we think we are, anyway—we are indulging the hindrance of egoism. Ultimately, this *klesa* also arises from an ignorance, or disparity between perception and reality.

There are a great many things we are physically unable to perceive, which plays into our lack of understanding. Our eyes can only see a certain frequency range within the light spectrum; similarly, our ears can only hear a given range of sound. Along with missing the big-picture truth of a situation, we also misidentify what our highly limited sense organs tell us about the world. This egoistic point of view has us thinking that what we perceive and believe is the be-all and end-all of who or what we are. We act as if our own egoistic thinking *is* pure consciousness, when in truth the subtle essence of our true nature is barely perceptible within the cacophony of thoughts and all that we see, hear, and feel.

The Identity Center

What our yoga practice eventually teaches us is that there is a gap between who we think we are and who we truly are. We tend to identify with our personality attributes, appearance, talents, and other qualities, when our true essence is ineffable. In fact, the ways we tend to recognize ourselves can actually interfere with our awareness of our true nature.

This concept is reflected in the name of the *chakra*, or energy center, associated with ego and sense of Self: *manipura. Chakras* are an energetic construct based on the circulatory system of our "subtle body." Where thousands of energy meridians intersect, we find major and minor *chakras.* The energy body is discussed more later in this chapter when you learn about the layers of being.

The ego's energy center, located at the solar plexus, is associated with our personality and reason for being, along with determination and motivation. It is a prime harmonizing place of who we think we are and who we really are, or where our individual gifts meet our spiritual purpose. The solar plexus, as its name indicates, is also associated with the sun and element of fire. This is a fire of purpose, as just mentioned, and fire of purification, where we burn off egoistic impressions and unite with the creative Self. *Manipura* translates as "hidden gem."

Perhaps you hold the idea of your creative soul as the sparkle and color that's encased within your personality, aptitudes, and interests. The more we align with those true parts of ourselves—what we inexplicably came to this world with, free from external programming and our own tightly held beliefs—the more we allow ourselves to shine. The following practice supports you in aligning your material and spiritual selves.

Exercise: Yoga Posture Practice: Balance the Ego Center (*Manipura Chakra*)

Let this sample practice be a guide to your own exploration. Most of the postures listed below are energetically or archetypically aligned with the solar plexus associations listed above. There are no firm lines drawn around our interconnected *chakra* system. Each *chakra* has its own associations, for example the joy and love of the heart or clarity and insight of the third eye or creative feeling of the sacrum. *Chakras* are connected with one another as part of an energetic system and, like the body, their home cannot be parsed into separate, unrelated segments. Thus, you can play with this and other practices in this book.

What happens if you perform the same sequence with a different intention or *chakra* focus, such as the root, throat, and crown? How about doing other posture sequences in this book guided by the solar plexus? If you wish to explore more about your *asana* practice and the *chakra* system, archetypes, or intention, see *The Pure Heart of Yoga* by Robert Butera.

Step 1: Warm up your body. You can do this by walking, swinging your arms and legs, or dancing a little soft shoe. Once you are ready for *asana* practice, face the long edge of your mat. Hold the lower body still, as if you were on the beach buried in sand up to your hips. Initiate movement from the solar plexus as you revolve your torso methodically from side to side. Hold your arms out to the sides, palms up or down, and look around with the head and eyes in the same direction you are twisting. You may experiment with linking the movement to the breath, so each time you twist you inhale then exhale back to center, or vice versa. Now, face the front, raise your arms overhead, and side bend left and right. Be sure to initiate the movement from the solar plexus and stay connected to what is happening at the base of your rib cage (solar plexus area) in the front and back of the body. You may practice the following sequence all on one side, then switch to the other or, as indicated in the instructions, do each pose on both sides before moving on to the next posture.

Step 2: Warrior II (*Virabhadrasana II*)—Still facing the long edge of your yoga mat, step your legs from two to three feet apart. Turn your left foot ninety degrees, so your toes and knee point to the left short edge of the mat. For balance and in order to keep your whole foot on the mat, your right foot may also angle inward (toward the left short edge of the mat) roughly fifteen degrees. Keep your chest/back facing the long edges of the mat as your arms stretch out to each side (left and right short edges of the mat), hands at shoulder height. Gaze over your left hand and bend into the left knee, keeping that knee above or behind the left ankle. Keep the right leg straight. Feel the fire of confidence warming you from that sunny center as you press strength through your legs and hold your core firm. Be aware of strength and confidence, holding the pose for thirty seconds up to three minutes. Repeat on the other side. Remain aware of the effects of these movements on *manipura*.

Step 3: Exalted Warrior—From Warrior II posture, shift into a backbend. First, revolve so that your chest now faces your bent (left) knee and the short edge of your mat. You may need to adjust your feet wider (imagine standing on railroad ties) for balance. Reach your left hand up, keeping the left knee bent, and lower your right hand toward your right leg. The right leg is straight and the entire right foot presses into the mat. Your intention moves from being one of forward-focused determination to that of exaltation and gratitude. Imagine connecting your personality to the divine cocreator and lift your solar plexus forward and up. Spread this opening sense upward and downward from that centered point. Repeat on the other side.

Step 4: Humble Warrior—Next, still in a Warrior base with your chest facing your bent left knee, interlace your fingers behind you or grip your front thigh for support as you twist toward it and fold forward, bringing your head toward the bent left knee. As you bow, imagine surrendering your ego to divine perspective. Feel humbled and soothed by the great mystery of creation. After a few breaths, rise carefully and repeat on the other side.

You may end the practice there or continue on with a mind-quieting technique. The more we practice quieting our mental chatter and changeable emotions, the better we are able to sense the voice of the true Self. The following exercise allows you to explore the subtle differences between your mind and your creative soul.

Exercise: Mindfulness Practice to Transcend the Ego

Spend the next two to thirty minutes moving through this mindfulness practice. Remember that your ego may resist the process: your mind may become jumpier, your emotions might unsettle, you may wonder about the point of it all or feel like you are wasting time. You might not "get it." Those are all normal reactions. Don't dwell on them. All you have to do is watch the play within your mind and body; just because it exists does not mean you need to act upon it in that moment (or at all).

Step 1: Settle into a comfortable standing or seated position. I recommend the latter because lying down typically leads to falling asleep and missing the final steps of the exercise. As you settle, notice how your body feels. Where are your muscles tight and where are they loose? Which parts of you rest into gravity and which ones resist? Acknowledge pain, restfulness, and any other notable feelings without trying to change anything.

Step 2: Allow your awareness to shift to your breath. Again, do not change it, simply witness how your body moves the air. Notice if the breath itself seems to adopt a pattern, depth, and timing.

Step 3: Witness the thoughts that you are thinking. You don't have to change or act on these, either. Simply notice the content and quality of the things your mind thinks of. Do not judge these things; no matter what they are, these thought patterns contain a great deal of information for you. Watch them flow and also acknowledge any emotions that may flow alongside them.

Step 4: Move to a more subtle layer and notice the part of you that is doing the noticing. Connect to this object witness self. Does this connection to the witness create some distance between your sense of Self and the thoughts that move through your mind?

Step 5: The discerning internal witness resides close to your creative soul. Invite the presence of your spiritual Self to join the witness. Another way to think of this is to turn your witness away from the externally driven inputs of body, breath, and mind; instead turn inward to the essential Self. Although you may not be able to tell if you are actually watching your true Self or simply attending another layer of your mind, it is enough to intend to perceive your deepest Self. Once that part of you knows you are paying attention, it will reveal itself more and more clearly. Ask your creative Self to reveal some form of support or encouragement to you. Your ego may jump in and scoff at this idea or what is revealed—it can even interfere with transmission—but all you have to do is trust yourself and ask again. Remain open to what appears, even if you don't get it or it seems weird.

Step 6: Carry this encouragement from your creative Self with you. Witness your thoughts again without trying to change them, only this time allow the support of your essential Self to color those thoughts. Shift your awareness to your breath and, similarly, allow the breath to find its own depth and pace while you intend to breathe the encouragement. After a comfortable number of rounds, bring your awareness to your body and feel the presence of spiritual support within your physical self. Perceive how this divine creative presence can exist through all your layers of being.

Step 7: Acknowledge what you noticed as you moved your awareness inward from body to breath, mind, witness, and soul. What were some reoccurring themes, sensations, beliefs, or emotions? When you connected with your creative Self and received encouragement and support, did you notice different things as you came back out through the same layers? Did the layers themselves impact one another? For example, did your breath affect your thoughts? Did your thoughts affect your body? Using pastels, sand, or a tub full of water, express the inward journey. Use the nebulous nature of these media to relate to the interconnectedness of your own inner layers. In the following section, we relate those layers to ancient yoga philosophy.

What You're Made Of

During that exercise, you traveled through five layers of existence. A number of *Upanishads* (ancient Indian writings espousing the nature of the soul) speak of humans as possessing five layers, or sheaths (*koshas*). This concept is not so foreign when we consider the modern body-mind-soul paradigm. The *Upanishads* indicate that the body is home for the breath-energy (*prana*), and within that is the mind (our wandering thoughts, sense impressions, passing emotions, etc.). Within the mind is the more subtle intellect, which houses our entrenched beliefs, programming, and some *karmic* impressions but is also able to discern between matter and spirit. Most subtle of all, within the intellect, is the "bliss sheath" (*anandamaya kosha*). The true, creative Self shines from this place through the other layers of our being.

When we get caught up in the level of the body, energy, mind, or even the discerning intellect, we have fallen prey to the hindrance of egoism. Similar to the *chakra* system, the *koshas* are interconnected, synergistic layers. Please remember that the breath is part of the body and the mind is a part of them both. The intellect can be seen in those layers and spirit radiates through all of them. The following exercise helps you befriend the power of intellect's discernment and steer your mind in the direction of the subtle, creative soul.

Exercise: Expressing, Exploring & Connecting to Your Craft

When we reflect upon the yoga philosophy of the *koshas,* we see that there are many layers to who we think we are. In the previous mindfulness exercise, did you notice how your thoughts and feelings changed depending upon which layer your mind was set to? This is experiential evidence that our point of view can quickly change what we believe and how we relate to the world. Try this adaptation experiment:

Step 1: Pick a creative outlet that is important to you. It can be something simple, such as cooking, cleaning, or coloring, or bigger tasks, such as screenwriting, composing, or carving. Hold the tools of your trade, such as spoons, pens, staff paper, or whatever they may be. (If you don't have the necessary instruments yet, just imagine yourself with them.) Notice, without trying to change anything, the thoughts, emotions, breathing patterns, and bodily responses that are present as you interact with these creative instruments. Set the tools aside for a moment and express the layers of what came up for you. What did you observe within yourself? You may use sculpture, drawing, or writing; whichever medium you select is to be used, on a fresh sheet or with new materials, in each of the following steps of this exercise. When your expressive work is complete, give yourself a few deep, clearing breaths.

Step 2: Hold the implements again. Move your body as an artist in this field would wield the instruments or mime using them. In what ways does this feel freeing and natural? In what ways is it foreign or ominous? Where is there tension or relaxation in your body as you pretend to use the tools? How is the depth, pace, and location of your breath? What thoughts are with you? Are they similar or do some thoughts contradict others? Can you discern the nay-sayers from your authentic voice? What emotions are present? Allow yourself to feel their range. Set the implements aside so you can use the same expressive modality you chose in step 1 to express what you observed here in step 2. Take a few deep breaths and let this step go.

Step 3: As you hold the tools of the trade again, imagine the energy a true artist in this field embodies. You may call to mind a mentor or an artist in this field you admire or resonate with. You may picture a version of yourself living as this kind of artist. Feel this way of being fill you. Breathe the breath of such an artist! After a couple of minutes imagining, embodying, and breathing, express your observations with the same medium. Take a few deep, natural breaths to clear yourself before moving on to step 4.

Step 4: Hold the instruments again or set them on a table in front of you and rest your hands upon them. Gaze at your hands holding or touching these tools. Fill your mind with thoughts of their use, of creating with them. Allow your gaze to be a soft focus—it may even blur—as your mind absorbs a sense of internal and external relationship with these tools. What emotions arise? After gazing and contemplating for a couple of minutes, set the tools aside and express the thoughts and mental impressions you had as you gazed at the instruments in your hands, then cleanse yourself with conscious breath.

Step 5: Imagine this craft has a guide, patron saint, or great master that you can pray or plug in to. In whatever way is meaningful to you, whether it's through pure imagination, writing a letter, having a conversation, contemplating, meditating, or some other form of reaching out, rest in the pure, kind company of wisdom and mastery. If your mind wanders, simply bring it back to your chosen manner of connecting to a great awareness and support of your craft. Sense the presence of a compassion-ate teacher who has practiced this craft for many years. Imagine that consciousness and discernment. It may take a few minutes to connect to this idea. Spend a few more exploring the insights that may be available. Then, express what you may have learned about how a master thinks or acts. Be creative!

Step 6: Bring the tools close to you and imagine that you have been working with them for years. They feel so comfortable in your hands it is almost as if they are a part of you. Encounter them as a familiar comfort. Feel at once enthused and relaxed by them. Imagine yourself a wizened old master of this art as you move and play with the implements. When you are ready, express this experience in the same medium you have been using throughout the exercise.

Step 7: Set your first expressive work, from step 1, next to the last, from step 6. In what ways are they similar? How do they differ? Did shifting the layer of focus also shift your per-spective or experience about becoming this type of artist? In what way? Did it feel different in your body, breath, thoughts, emotions, or sense of Self?

Revisit this exercise any time your ego gets too noisy and judgmental. This exercise is a practice to regain confidence, spiri-tual support, and connection to the legacy of your craft. When we are humble, there is room to make mistakes and spend time learning about our craft before expecting it to come out well. The following externally driven exercise also helps you connect to your creative Self.

Exercise: Power Songs & Experimenting with Creating Life

This reflection-and-selection exercise supports you in gathering your inner sensibilities together, drawing them near, and applying them to create a better life. Follow these steps to shed the ego-chatter and connect to a deeper sense of knowing and faith. Enjoy a game of creating life.

Step 1: There is a song (at least one) where every time you hear it there is a visceral impact. Your body responds: it needs to air drum, sing, or make silly faces; your feet want to tap or hands gesture; the music and lyrics make you feel seen and understood. Think of a song that makes you feel emboldened and strong. This piece of music should have an immediate and consistent effect on your state of mind, sense of Self, or perception of reality. It might shift your inner world because it reminds you of something or someone, it contains a lyric that touches you, or the rhythm/melody is unstoppable.

Step 2 (optional): If you can't think of a power song right away, don't worry. Now that you are curious about it, it will randomly show up in your world over the next few days. Keep an ear out! You can experiment this way if you already know your power song, as well. Notice how long it takes before you randomly encounter it in your everyday life. Some people believe the sooner it happens, the more you are living in alignment with your creative abilities. Consider that we create many aspects of our lives.

Step 3: As you listen to your power song, doodle silly sketches of the most outlandish things that are truly possible for you. You might come up with a cartoon about turning smog into diamonds, draw stick figures building wells outside African schools, or sketch yourself at your own book launch or opening night gala. Creativity and prospects come in all forms. Anything is possible for you.

Step 4: Come up with little experiments to create your ideal life. What happens if you intend to find change on the sidewalk, bump into an old friend, or catch a string of green lights? How about when you wish for a rainy day, a political outcome, or someone's health to improve? It might be important, on this path of egoism, to understand what is ours, what is not ours, and what requires a community effort. Power songs and conscious creation connect us to our creative soul and so can the following exercise.

Exercise: Dance Party

Dance parties are important. They uplift us, offer whole-health benefits to many of the body's systems, and help blow off steam. Most dance parties happen in the living room; the kitchen is a close rival for dancing space. I have even heard that some people *go out* dancing—a rare event for introverted or busy people. Practice the following exercise often and with joy.

Holding the idea of your multilayered Self, put on your power song from the previous exercise, or some other catchy ditty, and let each layer of your being express itself through movement. You can systematically let each chorus and verse explore a layer, ensure that you are moving through all five consistently, or let each *kosha* decide when it wants to express itself as you trust the process. Remember to play with height, interacting with earth and sky, and move in all directions (ensuring there are no obstacles nearby).

Return to this exercise any time you need to move, get inspired, or shake off the stress of the day.

Now that you have explored your I sense, let's look at some of the more apparent ways the obstacles hinder the connection with your creative true Self. Seeking what we want and avoiding what we don't seem like natural aspects of the path to self-realization. The trick is discerning what level of self the desire or disgust is coming from: egoism or truth. The following chapter investigates how externally driven choices hinder true connection.

Chapter 4
Toward & Away

PART OF MY SPIRITUAL and creative lifestyle involves seeking wisdom from books. I have studied religious texts for more than half of my life and, as a philosopher, bookworm, and student of humanity, also derive meaning and guidance from the fiction I read. Sometimes I need a quick refresher or answer from my books, so I turn to favorite verses or simply ask a question and open to a random page, paying keen attention to the personal significance of the first sentence that jumps out.

There was one year where I held the *Bhagavad Gita*, a traditional yogic text, close at hand. To my great amusement, no matter what question I asked or which page I turned to, the *Gita* responded with reminders about "nonattachment." Never the same sentence twice, mind you. I must have found nearly every time that translator wrote the word "nonattachment" ... It is one of the main themes of the *Bhagavad Gita*.

Nonattachment is central to any enlightened or creative path. In order to choose what is right, we often have to let go of what we want or what is easy. It is so hard to release our selfish desires that almost half of the five main hindrances center on that very theme. The obstacles of attachment (*raga*) and aversion (*dvesha*) create powerful disruptions in our peace of mind. Attachment is wanting, liking, or clinging, and aversion is not wanting, disliking, or avoiding. If we apply these principles specifically to our creative life, we can see how wanting a certain outcome from or appearance of our art can influence how much faith and enjoyment we apply to its creation. Being attached to or feeling dislike for certain outcomes, others' reactions, or a particular process is distracting and stressful. This chapter explores attachment and aversion while supporting you on a path of stilling this pendulum between desire and disgust through action and acceptance.

You may be thinking, "Shouldn't I move toward what I wish for and stay away from what I don't?"

In action, yes. But not in thought. Stay present with what is; presence immediately limits most of the *klesas'* impact upon your inner connection. The compulsion to move toward or away from something disrupts the mind because it is not a true path. Peaceful, measured action based on the inspiration of the creative soul has a very different sense than our petty attachments and aversions. In the beginning, especially if you don't have much practice quietly watching your inner world, it can be difficult to discern a true calling from a compulsion. Try the following exercise to experiment with experiencing the subtle difference.

 Exercise: Discerning Truth from Compulsion

Wise ones from many spiritual traditions believe that our true, creative Selves are continually communicating with us. Through subtle feelings, passing thoughts, and even "coincidences" in the world around you, spirit is passing messages. Consider the possibility that tuning out or ignoring these subtle cues is a form of self-betrayal. Read on to experiment with cultivating a more truthful communication.

Step 1: Think of a want that you have but know is not good for you, for example a certain relationship, lots of cookies, or cocaine. Watch the wanting happen within you to get as clear as possible about how it feels to want this.

Step 2: Grab an old magazine and rip out images that appeal to you. Spread them out in front of you and arrange them in ways that seem to tell stories or convey ideas. Notice the many different ways the images relate to each other (or don't): color, theme, mood, shapes, etc.

Step 3: Why did you choose those images? You may not know the answers. Our creative inspiration flows from great mystery. No need to be "attached" to knowing. Notice how you feel when you look at them.

Step 4: It is likely that the harmful desires do not flow from the creative Self while the imagery is a mirror to a truth within us. Considering the feelings you noticed in step 1 and step 3, was there a difference? How were the qualities of emotions similar or different? What was different in your body? Your breath? Your thoughts? Write down the clues that indicate you are receiving guidance from your creative Self.

The true, creative Self is wise but subtle. On the other hand, attachments and aversions arise from our programming or past pain. As you continue this journey of removing the obstacles between everyday-you and your creative essence, you will enjoy a greater self-knowing and sense of balance in day-to-day living.

Balancing Action & Acceptance

Our attachments and aversions are typically created out of past experiences. The *Yoga Sutras* says these wants arise from things seen or heard about previously. They are a *predetermined* path. "I like these. I don't like those." Such points of view are programmed by our existing biases; we could say that is another form of *karma* playing out. Awareness, action, and acceptance are simple ways to break through these automatic reactions.

Attachment is clinging. We seek out what we think we want. In modern society, we are taught that attachment is a normal, even desirous, approach to life. However, the wise understand that seeking what we do not have is a path to misery and a clear obstacle to union with the creative soul.

The *Bhagavad Gita*, in its poetic approach, teaches that it is our duty to act in accordance with the truth of our soul, but we have no right to the results of that action. If we act with a narrow hope for a specific end, that attachment to a predetermined outcome creates *karma* and squelches creative possibilities. If, on the other hand, our choices arise from the calling of our soul and we act for action's sake, not outcome's sake, the intentional awareness helps neutralize *karma*. Acknowledging the meaning of the action itself, no matter how it turns out, allows the soul to shine through both actions and outcomes. Trusting the call of the soul and ourselves in the action, we can accept the end result. Trust yourself, do your best, then let it go.

Aversion is the mind, and by extension our actions, repelling something unwanted. It is sometimes called an attachment to hatred or disgust. Consider a person with cleanliness obsessions. This person appears to be grossed out by germs, but if we examine the state of mind, we see that it is wrapped up in thinking about those microbes. Even though one tries to get away from being dirty, the filth collects in the mind continuously. By removing the obstacle of aversion, we move beyond the readily available option ("I don't like/want that") to the transcendent option of acceptance. This latter option is not about changing the situation itself; rather, it is about how we interact with and perceive the reality. Act prudently, without attachment to the results—even if things turn out not how you want. By holding an intention of acceptance (or other spiritually based concept), we change our thoughts and release the hindrance. The following exercise gives you some practice in releasing attachments and cultivating acceptance.

Exercise: Letting Go of Attachments

This exercise helps you name the losses that go along with living more creatively. Be as specific as possible about the things you will miss (attachments) when you connect to your creative Self more deeply.

Step 1: Rest comfortably and, in as much detail as possible, imagine yourself living more creatively. See how you spend the average day. When do you get up/go to bed? What do you eat? Who do you associate with? When and what do you create? How does it feel? Are there other things you do with your spare time? You may draw on past attempts to follow your creative essence or completely make up a scenario. Notice how this ideal creative life is different from your current one.

Step 2: What losses come with living more creatively? What do you have to give up or let go of? What habits must change? What do you not have time for now that you are dedicated to self-expression and creative living? Notice what is lost when you don't have these things anymore. Pay careful attention to how that feels. You may choose to express these potential losses through movement, imagery, or sound.

Step 3: What are you not willing to let go of or change? Be truthful now, even if you think you "should" be able to release it. Write these habits down. If you acknowledge what you are not ready to let go of, when it appears as an obstacle you can smile at it and either carry it with you or find a way around it. Do you see how this is also a form of acceptance? Imagine these habits as objects you carry with you through your creative life, as imagined in step 1.

Step 4: If you continue holding on to this habit or lifestyle choice, what are the potential costs of keeping it for the next five years? For each of the habits or lifestyle factors you recorded in step 3, record the "Potential Costs" on a new sheet of paper with that heading. Visualize yourself attempting to set it down and notice, five years later, what the costs of letting go are. Imagine yourself holding it for another ten years and the effects of continuing this habit. What happens if you attempt to set it down then? How about twenty, thirty, or fifty years down the road? For each of these future visualizations, record any additional potential costs, as well as why it is difficult to release these things. Continue accepting yourself, your habits, and your desires/dislikes.

Step 5: For each potential cost, on a new piece of paper write an affirming, healthy statement to counter it. Destroy the Potential Costs page, feeling the new affirmations or uplifting beliefs instead.

Step 6 (optional): Envision the version of yourself from step 1 standing alongside the you in fifty years who is still carrying these items. Imagine a conversation between the two of them. Does your creative Self have reasons to let any of the habits go? If the part of you carrying the stones is willing to release any of them, perceive yourself naming and throwing each one away. Notice the space and lightness that is created when this obstacle is flung off. You may decide to go to a nearby body of water, name stones for your attachments, and enjoy the satisfaction of tossing them safely and legally into the water.

Step 7 (optional): If you chose to release any of the habits, how were you able to do it? What feeling or belief made it possible? Is there anything you are willing to let go of right now? Then let it go! It's okay. Accept that it just doesn't mean that much to you—or that something else is more important—and let it go completely. If there are many, you may wish to pick just one, master its absence, then move on to the next.

Through the course of this exercise you had the chance to discern what are truly obstacles, things you need to let go of, and what are aspects that you do not wish to release (even though "on paper" they may not be best for you). You can come back later and add to that list as you continue the journey. Realize there may be other things that, even if you don't like it, you aren't ready to set down yet. That's okay. Ultimately, the effect of those things, and what it takes to release them, may be a deep source of inspiration for your creative endeavors.

Now that you have some practice letting go of what you don't need (even if you want it), you may be ready to face some of your addictive tendencies. We all have them; some of us to a greater degree than others. Continue accepting yourself as you read through the section on addictions and notice how it relates to various areas of your lifestyle and beliefs.

Addiction: Aversion Hiding in Attachment

Addictions are sometimes known as unhealthy attachments. Although we think of addictions as attachments to the substance of choice (alcohol, drugs, caffeine, sugar, salt, shopping, sex, love, exercise, etc.), addictions actually reveal aversions. Most people are not indulging in unhealthy behaviors because they enjoy them, even though a pleasurable experience is part of it. Rather, addictions get us away from what we don't want to feel or experience: loneliness, anxiety, depression, etc. Thus, addictions tend to be more about aversion—moving away from uncomfortable feelings—than they are attachment. The impulse to seek the "good feeling" addictions temporarily bring is really a distaste for something deeply painful. However, we tend to become so obsessed with the object of our addiction that it helps us avoid the underlying aversion completely. We don't feel the pain when we are high on wine, sugar, sex, gambling, shoes, cleaning, etc., nor do we feel the pain during the come-down, nor while repetitively seeking the addictive substance or behavior.

Creative people tend to be prone to addictions. This may be because of a tendency to be more sensitive to the world and our own emotions (think of the classic "poet's soul"), because it is harder to fit into society with so many outside-the-box perspectives (which leads to a sense of isolation), or because of a false identification with the wounded artist archetype (e.g., Hemingway, Van Gogh). Whatever the reason, it is beneficial to explore the role of addictions—facing the aversions and unwinding the attachments—as we connect to the creative essence.

When we are caught in addictive patterns, there are many paths to freedom. You may seek help from a physician, alternative healthcare practitioner, counselor, or rehabilitation program. In addition to professional support (which this book cannot replace), you can work with the following yoga therapy technique. This technique looks at identifying and working with the unmet need and practice of channeling pain into personalized expression. Remember that fundamental attitude of acceptance as you move through the next exercise. This exercise can be especially powerful if you apply it *during* moments when the addictive urge is upon you. Facing our addictive tendencies, and choosing a creative outlet rather than ignoring or tearing down our authentic knowing, is an uplifting and potent way to harness creative power.

Exercise: Soothing the Unmet Need

When we feel compelled to turn to something outside of ourselves to meet an internal need, especially if that external substance causes some form of harm (on the lungs, liver, relationships, finances, etc.), we repeat *karma* rather than healing the needy place. This exercise helps you identify and begin to meet a deep, hidden need. Remember that when we express/create, we are releasing what was hidden inside.

Step 1: Notice what happens in your body when you are triggered to play out an addiction. Acknowledge the breathing pattern and thoughts/feelings that go along with being triggered. When you become very adept at this, you will begin to notice signs and symptoms minutes, hours, and even days before the acute addictive behavior is activated. If, on the other hand, you are not in touch with that sense, flag or dog-ear this page and set the exercise aside until a more relevant time.

Step 2: Represent the visceral, energetic, and emotional patterns with color and shape. I recommend using crayons. If it is difficult to draw, for whatever reason, switch to using your non-dominant hand or even your teeth to move the crayon over the page. This expressive process will likely intensify the feelings during the time they move out of you.

Step 3: Use these intensified feelings to focus on a specific need crying out from within you. If you feel despair, you may need connection, hope, or gentleness. If you feel angry you may need to be heard, acknowledged, or reassured. If you feel lonely you may need touch, warmth, or a friendly ear. Write the need down. Don't worry if you aren't sure it's the "right" word or feeling. You can repeat this exercise as many times as you wish. For now, trust the word(s) that is/are arising.

Step 4: On a fresh sheet of paper, use color and form to express soothing the need. Let your body (even if it's your non-dominant hand or teeth) move with the quality that helps meet the need. Take as much time as you need. You may even repeat this step a few times.

Step 5: Note the sense that came through your body, breath, thoughts, and emotions. What was the quality that helped meet the need? Write it down next to where you wrote the need itself. If there were multiple qualities, please do record them all.

Step 6: Review the soothing drawing(s). Notice the effect on your physical, energetic, and emotional self. Quiet your mind as you regard the externalized representation of soothing. Allow whatever feelings arise to wash over you without attachment or aversion—simply witness and let go as you allow this expression from your creative soul to bring solace.

Step 7: Settle into a meditative or relaxation posture with your soothing image nearby. Bask in the comforting feeling that meets the unmet need for as long as possible. If you fall asleep, all the better to process through this deeper layer. Notice that even if your solace involves others, your emotions, thoughts, and beliefs are *within you*. Trust yourself to cultivate and feed your wounded self this deep, soothing quality. When you imagine the soothing, it is fully present within you. This is the power of your creative soul.

Step 8 (optional): While holding the intention/quality that helps meet the need, dispose of the original drawing. Let this process symbolically represent letting go of that layer of pain.

This exercise guided you to harness your creative soul so that unmet needs could receive what they require. We often think that we need something from someone else in order to let go of past pain. The reality is that if they were going to give that to us, they probably would have already; we could carry this pain forever, waiting for someone else to free us. Instead, realize that everything you need is already within you. No matter how attached you are to an outcome or the amount of aversion you feel toward certain emotions/circumstances, the power of your creative essence is stronger. You are a force of nature. By cultivating the qualities that support your own healing and expressing both the pain and the soothing, you are on a strong path to recovery—by your own independent choice.

Attachment and aversion alter our peace of mind. Compulsions to move toward or away from what we think we know disrupt our inner balance. Feelings of desire and disgust are obstacles between us and the true Self. Continue choosing to connect to your creative Self when you notice a pressure to get or get away from anything. As soon as you accept the moment as it is, your creative mind will rule your perceptual senses. A wealth of inspiration may flow through that open space; creative opportunities abound! Go ahead and move toward what you want and away from what you don't and let the mind stay present, outside of the outcome. Fear of the ultimate outcome is the topic of the next chapter.

Chapter 5

Fear

THE FINAL OBSTACLE BETWEEN the creative soul and our personality is known as "fear of death" (*abhinivesa*). This may sound at the same time highly common, as most folks don't want to die, and extreme, as we are not continually fearing death in everyday life. Think of it this way: when we resist change in life, we often have a list of rationalizations why. The yogis might suggest we could find a fear of death at the bottom of every rationale, whether moving on from a job, ceasing smoking, or starting a new routine. It is not that we are afraid such changes will literally kill us; rather, when we embark upon anything new, we face the unknown, just as death is an unknown. Furthermore, the familiar will die. These are frightening prospects, indeed. This chapter provides yoga philosophy and yoga therapy practices to help you transcend fear.

Exercise: Facing & Moving Beyond Fear

A common way to move beyond fear is to face it. If you are caught in a nightmare of being chased, you master the dream when you stop running and look at what is bearing down on you. This exercise gives you the chance to look at your nightmare scenarios and realize you *can* face them. Note that steps 3 and 4 can be powerful and you may wish to set them aside if you are in a psychologically difficult place. As always, trust and care for yourself; seek the support of your loved ones and professionals whenever needed.

Step 1: Take a few deep breaths or perform a quick mindfulness scan of your body, breath, thoughts, and feelings. Next, complete the following sentence by listing as many ideas as you can in one minute. It's okay to repeat yourself and be completely irrational. It's also okay to write down your genuine, deepest fears: *If I indulged in more creativity, terrible things could happen, such as* _____.

Step 2: Breathe deeply or perform a mindfulness check-in. Complete the following sentence using images in crayon. You may scribble or endeavor to draw pictures that represent the answers arising from within you. *Being creative is risky because*

_____.

Step 3: Clear yourself again with breath or mindfulness. Complete the following sentence by responding in nonverbal vocalizations and gibberish: *If I live a creative life, I am sure to* _____. Make an expressive list of what could happen, using only nonsense sounds and whatever gestures and movements are relevant to that speech.

Step 4: Pause and notice the sensations that linger within you after that gibberish expression. These kinds of vocalizations often unleash a wealth of emotional energy. With whatever music you wish, or none at all, dance out the feelings that gibberish brought up. For deeper impact, continue expressing yourself vocally as you move.

Step 5: Be kind with yourself. Nonverbal and bodily practices can be very intense. Care for yourself now by reclining and nourishing your senses: indulge in a bubble bath, diffuse essential oils, stream songs featuring your favorite instrument.

This exercise gave you the opportunity to knock some of your fears loose. Now that you are facing them, your courage will rise up in equal measure! The following yoga posture sequence can help you embody the resilience, vigor, and hopefulness required to act in the face of fear.

 Exercise: Yoga Posture Practice: Intentional Poses for Courage

Ensure you are sufficiently warmed up and prepared for strength and movement before beginning the following sequence. Throughout the yoga poses, hold the intention to face and smash through your fears. Different people require different qualities to make this happen for themselves. Apply focus to the intention that fits you best right now.

Step 1: Child's Pose (*Balasana*)—Bring yourself to the mat on your hands and knees position. Settle your seat toward your heels, with the top of the feet on the ground. Lean forward over your thighs to rest your forehead either in your palms, on stacked fists, or to the mat. If your forehead is on the ground, you can reach your arms on the floor overhead or alongside your torso and legs. You are curled up now. Knees may be together or apart. Allow mental busyness to drain out your forehead into the earth. Feel yourself curved as a fetus in a loving womb: totally warm, safe, and wanted. The root of courage is self-worth and personal standards. People are so glad you exist. You are a perfect creation. Bask in this for as long as you wish.

Step 2: Cobra Pose (*Bhujangasana*)—Lie down on your abdomen. Place your palms beneath your shoulders. If back comfort allows, bring feet and legs together so your body represents a sleek tube. (Imagine the same tube if your legs and feet are hip-width apart.) As you inhale, imagine a glorious king cobra: calm, focused, mesmerizing. The next time you breathe in, roll up your face and chest like a powerful cobra rising. Do not rely on your hands to push you and keep your snake belly on the ground. Lift your blazing eyes, lengthen the front and back of your neck, and be strong through the length of your body. As you gaze intensely forward, imagine your creative Self down a path in front of you. See this expressive, contented version of yourself in the act of creation. Notice the obstacles that stand between you and this version of yourself. They may appear as rocks, metaphorical symbols, or the literal things interfering with your creative journey. Trust what appears, then stare it down with your fiery snake eyes. Hiss. *Ssss!* Hiss again, louder. *HSSSSS!* As your tongue presses upward, feel your breath energy fill you, circulate through your body as it gathers strength, then release as a sound wave that shatters barriers. *HSSSSSSSSSS!* You may unroll the chest and face back to the mat, then roll up again to hiss away the obstacles. After performing this fortitudinous posture a few times, rest on your belly and cheek and enjoy the sensation of your breath against the ground.

Step 3: Plank/Half-Plank—After resting, turn your toes under (to the ground) and place your hands beneath your shoulders. Feel your mightiness as you push the earth away, moving through a push-up action to come into a plank or, if your knees are down and you are shaped like a ramp, a half-plank. Experiment with placing the effort in different parts of your body. What happens if your shoulders hold the posture? What if the work were in the chest or the back? Can the gluteal muscles in your bottom help hold you? Is there a difference between putting the effort in the smaller places (hands, pelvic floor, lips) and the bigger ones (quadriceps, pectorals, abdominals)? Acknowledge that you are strong in many ways.

Step 4: Crescent Moon—From Plank Pose, stabilize your upper body and, if possible, step your right foot between your hands. You may have to grab your foot and put it there or slide your entire body backward to get the right knee above its ankle. Once the knee is over the ankle, apply some downward pressure into the right foot. Place the left (back) knee on the floor. Hands may climb the right leg, resting on the thigh, or bring the palms together in front of the chest or overhead. Experiment with the strength and mobility of your pelvic area as you shift more weight to the front (right) leg. Secure your abdominals and begin to arch back slightly by making distance between your pubic bone, rib cage, and chin. Create space through the front of your spine as you arch upward, free and open as a crescent moon in the vast night sky. Remember your fearless intention and feel it filling the tremendous space within and around you.

Step 5: Lunging Twist—Straighten your spine so you are no longer in a back bend, then twist to the openness of your left side. If hands are on the front thigh they can help stabilize; otherwise, arms reach upward. When you are ready, maintain your strong base and revolve the torso toward the right side. Stay long through the spine and connected to a sense of strength and courage. After you have spiraled more of your intention into your being, untwist to center yourself and slowly bring your palms to the floor. Transition through step 3 and repeat steps 4 and 5 with your left leg forward this time. Be aware of any asymmetries, whether physical, energetic, emotional, or intellectual. One side may feel quite different from the other and stimulate various thoughts, feelings, or images as you continue on this path to aligning with courage. All you need to do is be aware—from awareness, the impetus for change occurs.

Step 6: Once you have repeated the actions on the second side, return to step 3 again. How does that posture feel different each time you return there? Isn't it incredible how quickly your body/energy/mind can change?

Step 7: Goddess Pose (*Deviasana*)—Find your way to standing up, facing the long edge of your mat, in a wide-legged stance. Yin energy is that of the feminine qualities, like a peaceful night: introspective, quiet, cool, receptive, fluid, creative. Apply these qualities to your intention of courage. You may imagine that resilient intention like a seed incubating in the earth or womb. Now sense that nurturing, protective space of the earth or womb in your own sacral area. Your feet can point straight ahead or on a forty-five–degree angle, right foot to right corner, left foot to left corner of mat. Begin to bend the knees out to the sides, doing your best to keep them in line with the ankles, not caving inward. Feel a sense of presence at the sacrum and the corresponding place in your low belly. Keep the torso upright, with a natural curve in your spine. Stretch your arms to the sides in line with the shoulders then bend the elbows so the wrists are above them, palms facing forward. Experience a sense of divine empowerment as you stand firmly rooted, holding a strong presence within yourself and all around. Continue connecting to your creative space and gestate your intention. You may straighten the legs and rest the arms along your sides as you return to standing, then lower back to *Deviasana* numerous times.

Step 8: Side bending postures are thought to encourage the fluidity of the sacral energy center. From Goddess Pose, play with side bending lightly each way. Hold the wide-legged, knees-bent position and right-angled arms. When you side bend, you may aim your elbows toward hips or knees, without needing to actually touch them. Be sure not to roll forward or backward; just bend a comfortable distance from side to side. Continue connecting to the sacral *chakra* and creating a vibrant intention to flow through your life.

Step 9: Center yourself and reach the arms overhead as you straighten your legs. Become long and tall. Then lower your arms, gaze forward, and keep your weight even between your right and left feet. Notice the effect of the intentional practice on your desire to move forward through fear and bravely connect to your creative essence.

Step 10: Create an expressive piece that conveys the after-effects. Post or revisit this piece as a means of keeping your intention vital and your courage strong. You can rely on these virtues when resistance and fear arise … most of the time.

The previous practice supports you in uniting your body, breath, thoughts, feelings, and creative Self. It is common to end an *asana* practice with relaxation. Although it isn't necessary, you may choose to practice step 2 of the following exercise as part of the previous one to round out your posture sequence.

Relaxation: A Yoga Therapy Key

Relaxation is a common aspect of yoga practice. Your weekly class teacher has probably told you that Corpse Pose (*Savasana*) at the end of class is a time to let go of any clinging worries and bodily tensions. The peaceful space allows the mind and body to integrate the benefits of practice. If you suffer from stress or anxiety, you may know the value of just a few minutes of targeted relaxation practice. It resets the autonomic nervous system, alters brainwaves, and promotes the body's healing resources.

These physiological effects have psychological counterparts. Our state of mind changes when we are relaxed. We are more receptive to new ideas and ripe for inspiration. We have more energy to proceed with what we envision and, because we are relaxed and content rather than pressured and fearful, we are more likely to realize the positive benefits of our creative process. Relaxation simultaneously helps us hold laser focus and keeps our minds wide open to flashes of brilliance.

The following exercise gives you a chance to play with the opposites that live within you.

 Exercise: Side-by-Side Comparison of Nay-Sayer & Creative Self

In this exercise we will place a creative, relaxed state next to an uninspired, tense one. As you engage your mind in creating these diverse ways of being, discern what, specifically, is the difference between them.

Step 1: Hold a paper plate or a piece of construction paper to your face and gently mark where your eyes and mouth are. Hold the paper over a table, no longer near your face, and cut holes where you made the marks. Cut holes in the same place on a second "mask." You can also use foam, clay, or purchase blank templates upon which to paint masks. We will get to these shortly.

Step 2: Rest comfortably. Be aware of your body settling, supported, and notice the deep, easy flow of your breath. Connect to the uplifted enthusiasm of your creative Self, like that feeling you get when a new idea strikes.

Step 3: After you have basked in that goodness for a few minutes, juxtapose that creative sense with the fears of your disconnected self. Notice what happens to your body, breath, and thoughts as you gather your doubts, resistances, and worst-case scenarios. What if the nay-sayers are correct?!

Step 4: Grab one of your mask templates and create the face of your uninspired self. You may use color, decorations, and facial expressions to denote that dry, bored, low-energy state.

Step 5: The second mask is to express your creative Self. It may be worth relaxing again and intentionally invoking that juicy freedom before creating its face. No nay-sayers live in *this* realm! Be as colorful, playful, and strange as you want.

Step 6: Set these masks beside one another and take some time to reflect. You may choose to create a third piece (in a different medium such as psychodrama, dueling string instruments, or a cartoon) that expresses the relationship between these two states. Keep the masks handy and use them to express resistance, accept relapse, or invoke inspiration as needed. You can wear one or the other of them to exaggerate, invoke, or exorcise interference.

In order to live into the vision of our creative Selves and become the person each of us uniquely is, we must transform our relationship with fear. Rather than allowing it to dictate our limits and choices, we can use it as a trigger for courage and possibility. Try the following exercise to promote courage every time your fear starts to get the better of you.

Exercise: Gathering Courage

Fear not only limits our connection to the true, creative Self but it also narrows our lives and potential joy. Revisit this exercise any time you catch yourself avoiding, making excuses, or feeling genuinely nervous about something.

Step 1: Name your fear(s) or the action you are afraid of taking.

Step 2: Name ten good things that could come of you moving forward or taking action. I wanted to tell you to name twenty but was afraid you wouldn't do it. Wait ... Did I say "afraid"? Name twenty things that could go well from you taking this fearful action. Name them out loud. *Louder!*

Step 3: As you list these positive possibilities, notice the effect on your tone of voice, breath, thoughts, and embodiment. Can you feel the presence of courage filling you as you build faith through this process?

Step 4 (optional): If, when you set these benefits beside the costs/your fears, you still do not wish to take action, it is time to accept yourself and all involved, let it go, and move on. Nurturing a desire you do not wish to take action on is a waste of your resources and talents. If the issue arises again, repeat step 4 or consider the following step.

Step 5: Do that thing (or the next step toward that thing) that you are afraid of. It may still scare you a bit, but you are ready to do it anyway. Courage isn't about not feeling fear, it's about being afraid and doing it anyway.

You can see how the fear of death or change is a highly limiting obstacle on our creative path. If we focus on what could go wrong, or what we may lose, then we are meditating on obstacles to enlightenment, rather than enlightenment itself. When we focus on possibility instead—"What wonderful things could happen?" "What if your dreams came true?"—we are already more aligned with our inner truth and higher potential. This chapter gave you insight and tools to face and transcend your fears so that you can live into your possibility, truth, and higher potential. Through naming your fears, moving with intention, observing an internal stadium of relaxation versus fear, and cultivating courage, you are now ready to face your deepest fears and proceed on the path of alignment with your creative Self.

Now you have explored the five main obstacles between the everyday you and your creative soul: ignorance, egoism, attachment, aversion, and fear of death or change. Revisit this section on the Path of Creativity anytime you are feeling deeply hindered in your self-expression or sense of inner connection. You will be amazed by how the chapters and exercises seem different each time, and yield different outcomes, because you yourself are different when you come back to them. May this book continue to support you in removing all that stands between you and the brilliant creator that you *are*.

Part 2
Accessing the Creative Soul

YOGA IS A JOURNEY to union with your true Self. My training as a psychotherapist, via expressive arts and yoga therapy, taught me the importance of working with the individual. Each person has a unique path to self-understanding; each voice is its own. Every one of us has our own truth and we can access it through yoga practices and creative endeavors.

Consider the possibility that, just as a *meditative* state bestows an enlightened sense upon us, so does a *creative* state. Some might say that the flow of creativity is meditation. Creativity unites us with the truth of ourselves. I suggest, then, that when we create we are in a state of yoga—we are enlightened!

Yoga tradition teaches five paths to enlightenment. We can follow those same five paths to connect to the creative Self. The five Paths to Self-Realization are:

1. *Karma*, the path of purpose, service, or work

2. *Raja*, the systematic eightfold path of meditation

3. *Bhakti*, the path of devotion and emotion

4. *Jnana*, the path of the intellect and realized wisdom

5. *Tantra*, the subtle embodied path of connection

In this section, you have the chance to experiment with all five paths to get your creative juices flowing. Play with these approaches and see which ones suit you best. This is a great chance to explore your motivation and process as a creative being. You may also dabble in this section any time you are feeling blocked, uninspired, or like it is tough to get going on a creative project. Self-discovery happens via expressive arts and yoga therapy techniques (dance, drawing, humming, writing, poses, breathing, meditation, visualization, chakra system, chanting, etc.). The following concrete creative projects, emphasizing methods from each of five paths, support your inspiration and self-discovery.

Chapter 6

Via Purpose

THE FIRST OF THE five paths we are exploring is the path of *Karma* Yoga. In this context, *karma* can be thought of as purpose, work, or service. Simply stated, the *Karma* Yoga creator *works at it.* Through a clear personal purpose, or intention, and via a four-prong approach to action, you can be in service to your true, creative Self.

Dharma: The Intention Behind Your Art

The Sanskrit word *dharma* translates as "duty" or "purpose." *Karma*, or the patterns of our actions, is guided by our understanding of the duty that underlies our work. When we begin with a clear purpose, our actions filter through that intention. Like a golfer visualizing the ball landing in the hole before taking the swing, the *Karma* Yogi visions purpose before starting the work.

Exercise: Your Creative Purpose (Dharma)

This exercise gives you a chance to explore your creative purpose. Reflect and clarify your potential identity as a creative person through personal vision and intention.

Step 1: Reflect upon why you wish to be more creative. How is it beneficial for you to connect to your creative essence? Do others benefit as well? In what ways does your creativity relate to your purpose in life? Do you believe you have a duty to express yourself through creative acts? Why?

Step 2: Set an intention. This can be a word, a feeling, or a hope to express something that you're working through right now... Whatever is meaningful for you. Let it be brief and simple; imbue it with emotional relevance. Bonus points for writing it down, drawing it, or creating a collage that represents this purposeful intention.

When we know why we're creating, we have connected to *dharma*; we've set an intentional purpose for the creative act which then guides us. Intentional action guides the work and its outcomes—it's part of the *karma*.

Acceptance: Allowing & Trusting

The first step on the Path of *Karma* Yoga is "Acceptance." When we are aware of our *dharma* as creative beings, it becomes easier to accept the creative task at hand. On the *Karma* Yoga path, we approach all work with equanimity. We do not resist a chore; rather, we see all work as a creative opportunity. A balanced, accepting mind is open to the imaginative potential in every moment and action. The first step in any job is acceptance that the job exists.

When we are specifically talking about your art, accepting the need to create may be easy: "I accept that I'm seeing pretty pictures and must paint them." Or "I accept that these characters' dialogues are in my mind and I must film or write them." Or "I accept the lyrics and melodies that waft through my conscious and play them out on my instrument." However, it is not always that easy. Sometimes our creative urges swell from the darker corners of our psyches and express thoughts and impulses we would rather not admit to. Maybe something painful seeks expression as a way of releasing from our inner world. We tend to be less accepting of these kinds of creative tasks.

Many creative types who cannot find inspiration or initiate artistic action are not accepting the internal or external task at hand. The following exercise helps you build tolerance to what may be within you, allowing more room for acceptance and, by extension, creative freedom.

Exercise: Working through Triggers to Accept Strong Emotions

Most times when we have strong reactions to sensory input from the environment, we have tapped into a larger issue. The larger issue is probably some old, deep-rooted pain that is a little too terrible to face head-on, so instead we respond to immediate triggers in our environment. We don't wail about our dad walking out when we were four, we just get irrationally angry when we smell hot dogs, the last meal we shared before he left. We don't seek counseling after an assault, we just leave the party whenever we smell a particular cologne. We don't talk about the embarrassment of throwing up in class, we just never eat pizza again. The following exercise helps you connect with a deeper level of feelings and process to a more secure level of awareness—and hopefully acceptance—of those emotional reactions.

Step 1: Think of a song you skip every time it comes on. No matter where you are or what mood you are in, you still won't suffer that one track. You hate it that much. (At this point I could recommend you revisit chapter 4 on aversion, but for now, let's continue with this hard-to-listen-to song.) Cue it up, but don't play it yet.

Step 2: Lie down on your bed or yoga mat and perform a few gentle movements to get in touch with your body and bring a sense of physical pleasure and relaxation before settling into a relaxed position.

Step 3: Play the song and remain connected to the thoughts, feelings, and images that arise as the first verse happens.

Step 4: After the first chorus, stand up and use movement to express the thoughts, feelings, and images that you observe as the song continues. These movements may also be informed by step 3. Let yourself go into the process, accepting the shapes, sounds, and feelings that occur. Dance with these shadow emotions.

Step 5: You may replay the song a few times, emphasizing either step 3 or step 4 to gain a greater understanding of the real reason you have an aversion to this particular creation.

By giving yourself the opportunity to examine and express your authentic reactions to this song, you offered acceptance to the situation. This was not an exercise to help find appreciation for something you previously disliked; rather, an opportunity to witness and allow your genuine feelings. The skill of acceptance will support your endeavors as a creative person. As you practice accepting your internal states, thoughts, and feelings as they are, you have more genuine materials to create with.

Concentration: Be With It

The second step on the Path of *Karma* Yoga is "Concentration." Once we accept what we are bringing with us to the creative act, we focus on it. Give yourself over to the creative task! When we concentrate on the artistic act itself, being with our breath, emotions, and the expressive modality, our meaning comes through more clearly. Sometimes we express things that are beyond words: the depth of our pain, the heights of our joy, the vast isolation of human existence, the subtle awe of nature … When we contact the ineffable in this way, we may have a habit of becoming calculating, judgmental, or analytical. In other words, the depths of our expressive potential trigger our resistance. We may lose focus when we encounter something deep and true.

The following exercise gives you a chance to induce concentration and practice in maintaining it throughout the creative act. It is also a relaxation activity that can be applied as a mind-quieting technique.

Exercise: Creating from the Meditative Mind

You may use this technique when your nay-sayers get too loud or you feel disconnected from a project. It is also a lovely self-soothing practice in times of stress.

Step 1: Sit in a comfortable, erect position with finger paints or chalks in front of you. Close your eyes and attune to the natural rhythm and pace of your breath. You need not change anything; simply focus on the sense of each in-breath, each out-breath, and any breaks between them.

Step 2: Call to mind a shape or color. If you are less visual, you may posture your body into a particular shape or make a specific sound instead. As you hold this image, posture, or sound, notice how it interfaces with your breath. When you inhale, what does it do? How about when you exhale? Does it change during the pauses between the breaths?

Step 3: Continue concentrating on the depth, rhythm, and quality of your breath as you open your eyes. Using your non-dominant hand, squirt the finger paints or begin creating shapes with the chalks. Allow the hands to work as an extension of the breath.

Step 4: Let your breath facilitate this process—no thinking! As you follow your breath, your nondominant hand or both hands swirl the colors in relation to the inhales, exhales, and pauses. If your mind wanders, bring it back to the link between breath and expression. Your hands are instruments of your breath.

Step 5 (optional): If you are an experienced meditator, you may bring mindfulness to this process, consciously observing the motion, breath, thoughts, and feelings as your hands express. If this added dimension of awareness is distracting to your process, leave it out.

When you are in the zone with your creation, no one needs to tell you to concentrate. You are under a spell. Time has ceased to exist and your personality sets itself aside. Many folks say they feel as if their art were creating through them. This is creative magic! It happens spontaneously; furthermore, when we practice concentration and stay connected to our breath and internal senses, we enter that zone of creative flow more frequently and readily.

Excellence: Getting Out of the Way

It's very challenging to give your complete, relaxed concentration to something and do a bad job. The third step of *Karma* Yoga—"Excellence"— arises from the previous two steps. Once we have accepted ourselves and the task and fixed our breath, bodies, and mind to it, excellence follows. Excellence in this context does not mean creating a critically acclaimed piece; what it means is realizing the ultimate truth of the moment. Trusting what is and not letting judgments, preconceived notions, or expectations interfere with the purity of the experience.

 Exercise: Excellence Is Doing Your Best: A Practice for Perfectionists

The trick to being excellent is to accept that each of us has our own "best." Even within ourselves, what is best one day might be better or worse on another day. "Excellence" is about doing your best in the moment, not about being better than yourself or anybody else who has done a similar thing. The following practice helps bring a broader perspective to the concept of excellence. Follow either a or b.

Step 1: Lay newspaper or a drop cloth over your creative space, then line up paper and crayons (a). Alternatively, you may settle in front of your musical instrument (b).

Step 2: (a) Blindfold yourself or (b) put on mittens or gloves.

Step 3: (a) Draw a picture or (b) improvise a musical solo. Be free with this. Enjoy all of it, even the missteps and frustrations.

Step 4: Reflect upon the work. What did you learn about your ability to be excellent? How can you accept yourself more completely the next time you do something creative?

Oftentimes when we work on a creative endeavor we hold the end in mind, not from the perspective of *dharma*, where our effort falls in line with a personally meaningful intention, but from the perspective of "outcomes," where we seek a specific result. In hoping for a particular ending, we lose concentration and interfere with the excellence of our process.

Consider the story of musical great Herbie Hancock, who once struck a "wrong" chord while backing up the incomparable Miles Davis. Instead of judging the experience or even doing what most professionals would have done and played on, Davis took the accidental chord as a cue and played a phrase that made it fit. When we trust what comes out in the moment and work *with* it, we meet the opportunity to transcend what was possible before that unexpected event.

Trust yourself. Get out of the way. Work with what comes up. Let excellence speak for itself. Failing that, remember that everything you create is a step in the direction of your personal masterpiece. Ultimately, the final product is far less important than the grounded awareness you bring to your process. What you come out with is a piece of yourself... and we ain't always pretty.

Nonattachment: My Truth Is Enough

Now that you have explored the first three steps of the fourfold action of creative work, it is time to let go of the outcome. That's right. You were Accepting, Concentrated, Excellent, and now I'm asking you to not be attached to the end result. The final step is "Nonattachment."

If you are putting yourself out there—submitting your poem to magazines, trying to sell your photographs, or attempting to get your paintings into a gallery—you have a specific outcome in mind, and it is challenging not to be attached to that. When you show your best friend a new drawing—"Look what I made!"—then it's your heart on a plate. How can you not be attached to how others receive it? Yet in order for us to remain enlightened in our creativity, we must trust the life of the art itself.

For each expressive piece you make, your creative process is a journey. Believe in the truth as it comes out of you, no matter how it ends up. Imagine that your creative Self is its own entity flowing out of you as an expression of your true Self. If it is true to you—if you accepted, focused, and did your best—there is no need to be attached to how it turns out or how others respond. It is your truth, and it is perfect.

 Exercise: Practicing Nonattachment by Showing Yourself

This exercise challenges you to practice nonattachment. It is a systematic process, so you may wish to flag this page and return to each step a week or two later. Otherwise, gather it all up and get it over with. Learn about yourself, journal the insights, and feel strong and proud. This one is not easy.

Step 1: Find something you made that isn't great. Maybe its balance is off, maybe an experiment failed, maybe it's just ugly. This piece would probably be rejected by critics but it means something to you. Show this piece to someone you care about, without defending or explaining it. "Look what I made!"

Step 2: Find something you have worked on that has potential, such as a poem that needs a few more edits, a song without a chorus, or a short film that is missing a scene. Put the finishing touches on it and ask for feedback from one of your artistic mentors.

Step 3: Find a finished piece. Go to a local small artists' gallery and ask to show it. If it is music, find an open mic night. If it's literature go to a coffee house and do a reading. Put yourself out there for the sake of practicing nonattachment.

Remember for each of these steps to refine your ability to let go of outcomes. Do not judge your end piece or others' reactions. Do not hope things go well. Simply know your intention and let outcomes be outcomes, without attachment.

Your personal purpose gives meaning to all of your jobs. Let life itself be a creative act. Rather than getting hung up on your art as solely a final piece of work, you are enriched by intention—imagination and artistry are personal growth tools and the act of creating is valuable. By taking emphasis away from the end result, the path of *Karma* Yoga gives you a truthful perspective on your creative endeavors and keeps you enlivened and encouraged through times when the end result may not align with your hopes.

The path of *Karma* Yoga may be repeated several times with the same creation. For example, you might need to Accept the level of editing your story requires, or Concentrate on where the light is as you place the final shading on your drawing. You commit to Excellence when improvising the solo of a piece you've practiced a hundred times. You cultivate Nonattachment on opening night. All the while, your sacred duty (*dharma*) guides your process.

For example, as a member of a community orchestra, I have a sacred duty. I am responsible to the other musicians in my section to play well so we sound good together. Similarly, I must be well-practiced so the conductor doesn't have to waste time at rehearsals isolating parts. I have a duty to the composer to understand the piece and convey the message/feeling to listeners. The duty to entertain the audience may be the greatest of all; however, I believe the greatest duty is to my creative soul, who wishes to be seen and to express through union with the orchestra.

Even if I have to play something very fast, in a key with many sharps, I must accept it before I can go further. Saying "I hate this piece" isn't going to get anyone what is best. From there, I concentrate on learning the notes and rhythms, in addition to how they fit together with what others are doing. I do my best to practice in a variety of ways to secure my learning, and when rehearsals or the big show happens, I am not attached to the outcomes, knowing that I did my best all along. Although the intention is to be brilliant, if it doesn't turn out that way it's okay. If I practiced, listened, visualized, stayed relaxed, etc., what else was there? Beyond my best, there was nothing else I could have done. If I learned something from my mistakes, I will do even better next time.

Whether *Karma* Yoga, or the path of purposeful action, seems like your authentic path or not, check out the next chapter for a systematic approach to connecting with your creative soul.

Chapter 7
Using a System

THE SECOND PATH WE will look at arises from the 2,500-year-old work the *Yoga Sutras*. The *Raja* Yoga path, or "royal" path, is for the psychologically inclined, who prefer a systematic approach to self-understanding and expression. If your best approach to making something happen is to *do it*, this path is for you. *Raja* Yoga is a systematic process of quieting the mind so that the ever-present, but still and quiet, inner truth can shine forth. The first three *sutras*, or "threads", that weave the tapestry of the royal path loosely state, "Now we shall discuss yoga. Yoga steadies the distortions in our body-mind complex, then the true Self unites with the personality."

The *Yoga Sutras* proceed to offer readers an eightfold system of cultivating enlightenment in everyday life. Through ethical and moral principles, movement, and steadying the breath, senses, and mind, each of us can discover the subtle bliss that is our true nature and express from that unending truth. In this chapter, I apply the *Raja* Path to the creative process. By following this eightfold systematic approach, you have the chance to access and unite with your inner creator and allow that quiet, sacred aspect of your nature to express creatively.

Don'ts & Dos

The first two limbs of the eightfold path give us lifestyle guidelines in the form of restraining (*yama*) violent actions and observing (*niyama*) pure ones. The very first thing it teaches is to restrain from doing harm through action, word, or thought toward others or ourselves. This principle of non-harm (*ahimsa*) guides the *yamas*, which also include truthfulness (*satya*), non-stealing (*asteya*), healthful direction of vital energy (*brahmacharya*), and non-coveting (*aparigraha*). Let's look at these restraints in reverse order and apply them to accessing your inner creator.

As you strive to live a creative life, you may notice yourself wishing your work came out more like your vision of it or as good as another creator's. Coveting abilities we have not cultivated yet or talents of another person causes us harm because we are focused on a sense of lack rather than appreciation and creative freedom.

Brahmacharya is sometimes translated as "celibacy" or "continence," because sexual energy is very powerful. Think of it this way: there is an animating force flowing through us, what the yogis call *prana*. We only have so much vital energy to dedicate to our lives, which is one of the reasons we find it hard to pick up the pen or paintbrush after a long day getting the children ready for school, working, making dinner, cleaning up, and playing with the kids and pets. Our vital energy has been spent. When we consciously choose where to dedicate our energetic resources, not only do we not waste it on stress and overwhelm, but we are also able to mete it out more appropriately.

Non-stealing may seem obvious on the surface—you are not a robber!—but think about all the times you have stolen joy, rest, and creative opportunities from yourself, whether from choice, busyness, or fear. It does not have to be that way.

Truthfulness is another one most of us think we follow very well; after all, we are not liars. However, most of us have some trouble expressing our truth. We hold in our feelings, thoughts, requests to have our needs met, and other expressions of intimacy. Expressing ourselves creatively is an excellent means of practicing truthfulness, as our art expresses deep and even divine truths from our inner realms. You may further explore the first, guiding, *yama* in the following exercise.

Exercise: Facing the Habit of Inner Harm

We may not always notice when we create harm. Be gentle with yourself as you explore the next exercise.

Step 1: Think of a time when you created something and showed it to someone who did not understand. Perhaps this person judged you or your work harshly. He may have offered unsolicited feedback. Maybe she just didn't get it. To get the most out of this exercise, choose a moment that still contains a little sting. As a result of that moment, what did you come to believe about your art or yourself as a creative person? For example, if the conductor of your grade school choir told you no one wants to hear you singing that loudly, you may have begun to believe that "No one wants to hear me" or "My voice is not good enough."

Step 2: Work with this belief. Write a stand-up bit about that moment, a comic strip, or a movie scene. Draw it or sing it through a kazoo. Free your self-expression around that moment that may have genuinely shut down some of your creative instincts.

Step 3: Now consider what the opposite of that belief is. The *Yoga Sutras* chapter 2, *Sutra* 33, teaches us that when a negative arises, its opposite is to be contemplated. To continue with our example, your opposite belief might be "I deserve to be heard," "I give myself the freedom to speak my truth," or "What I have to say is good enough." Once you have formulated your opposite belief, phrased in positive language, write it on a sticky note and place it in an area where you work or create. You may post multiple opposite, affirming beliefs based on many past experiences in as many areas as you wish while you reprogram your self-harming beliefs. It is recommended that you change them somehow every two weeks or so, otherwise you will stop perceiving them in your environment and rather than being helpful tools, they become part of the background.

Step 4: Create a work in the same modality as step 2 that expresses this new, non-harming belief. Practice it regularly or post it where you are sure to see it often.

Typically, our self-harming habits arise from past programming: beliefs instilled in us from society, media, and caregivers. It is unlikely that anyone intended for us to create and carry lifelong negative beliefs about ourselves; however, it is the nature of humans, especially young ones, to take others' opinions personally and to hold on to the worst while discarding the best. As you continue to grow as a creative being, these old points of programming will emerge. Repeat the above exercise to support yourself in releasing this inner violence and opening a more creative approach to self-expression, unhindered by the echoes of judgment.

The process of eliminating these harmful core beliefs might also be seen as part of the second limb, the observances (*niyamas*). Just as nonviolence guides the restraints, so purity governs the observances.

Purifying our minds of negativity and judgment is an aspect of the approach, along with purifying our bodies through lifestyle choices and purifying our environments by keeping things clean and orderly. That's not always an easy thing to ask of a creative. The following exercise gives you ways of working with your own organizational system.

Exercise: Purifying Your Environment

If you are a certain kind of creative person, you may function well in a chaotic environment. The thing is, even though it looks like a mess to others, you probably know exactly where everything is. This exercise helps you explore why you have chosen this organizational system and offers ideas about how to use your unique process to inform a purer workspace.

Step 1: Have a look at the space where you work/create. Are you satisfied with the appearance of this area? Is it conducive to your creative process? Do you feel inspired by it? Does it reflect who you are as a person and a creator? I am infamously messy. While I enjoy the freedom of no one telling me what to do, I also feel distracted and stressed by the disorderly stacks of all manner of papers, images, pens, and whatnot that encroach upon my workspace.

Step 2: Notice how you organize yourself. Are you a piler or a filer? Do you need to see everything or do you prefer to keep your materials and documents out of sight? Do you prefer to act on one task start-to-finish or dabble between various responsibilities? Write down what you notice about the organizational strategy (piles, cupboards, like-with-like, most urgent to non-urgent, etc.).

Step 3: As you observe how you organize your materials, you will notice that there is a comfort in it, even if it winds up looking messy. If you are unsure about how your approach may be comforting you, try doing the opposite and your discomfort will come up pretty quickly. When I purchased an organizational system for my office, it sat empty while I continued to strew my work on the desk and the floor. Eventually, I realized I was afraid that if I put things away they would disappear. A more rational way of stating that fear was that I would never find them again or would forget to work on them. (Guess what. Both of those things actually happened when I used the organizational system … a lot!) While it is true that I did not prioritize "purity" as much as I could have, it is also true that I needed to see my stuff and could not figure out how to solve the paradox of serving that purpose *and* putting my stuff away. Consider your situation: write down the fears, worries, or anxieties your organizational strategy may be soothing. Furthermore, what potential problems does it help avoid.

Step 4: Once you have some theories about why you are messy in the way that you are, think of how you can meet your needs *and* organize your area. This may involve stacking in- and out-boxes, alphabetizing or prioritizing your projects, or, as I did, getting a plethora of shelf and cubby systems and hiding them behind a single closing door.

This effort toward purity or cleanliness helps the mind rest, as each time we see a mess it lodges as a to-do in our minds and interrupts the freedom of creative flow.

The other four *niyamas* also support our creative life. Contentment (*samtosha*) supports us in accepting our situation as it is and welcoming creative impulses, no matter how the endeavor turns out. Effort (*tapas*) is important, as without disciplined action we do not progress our natural abilities and are often unlikely to finish the projects we begin. Any creative action could be an aspect of the fourth observance, self-study (*svadhyaya*), which is the study of uplifting works as well as obtaining self-knowledge. The practice of surrendering to a higher reality (*ishvara pranidhana*) is valuable as you explore your creative side because it puts us in the habit of accepting what comes our way, letting go of outcomes, and remembering that we do not always have a clear view of the grand design. We never know where our ideas may come from, how we might be able to use the unfortunate events in our lives, or how the pieces of our lives fit together to create a bigger picture.

In the big picture of our everyday lives, the first two limbs on the *Raja* Yoga path, Restraints and Observances, help give us a framework of intention and behavior. While the *yamas* teach us to restrain that impulse to harm (in its various forms), the *niyamas* impel us toward purity of the external and internal. If there is something to be said and we limit our self-expression, then by the nature of silencing ourselves we have caused harm. If we are living in a messy environment, our creative mind and being will also feel cluttered. Non-harm and purity guide the precepts of truthfulness, non-stealing, moderation, and non-coveting, along with contentment, disciplined effort, self-study. These guidelines for living create a climate where our minds are open and clear so that we are primed for inspiration and better prepared to carry out the creative acts.

Expressing through the Body

People often associate the third limb of the *Raja* Path, *asanas*, with the physical postures of yoga; however, we can elaborate this view to include our bodily health and relaxation. It is important to remember that the physical practice of yoga (*asana*) is much more than just poses.

Exercise: Learn to Communicate with Your Body

The body contains great wisdom and creative power. It can express. It carries feelings and insights. When we contemplate the many subtle ways we may harm ourselves, as we did in the previous section, we can see that not expressing ourselves over a long period of time can be a great harm. Holding in strong emotions can lead to a variety of physical complaints and even chronic ailments. The following exercise attunes you to bodily expression.

Step 1: Lie down in a comfortable position. If you suffer from a chronic condition, place your hands on an area of the body you associate with that issue. You may also touch a part of you that is acting up today or an area you wish to know more about.

Step 2: As you rest with your hands upon your body, feel yourself letting go. Imagine your tension draining away as your body surrenders into the support beneath you. There is nothing to resist; no parts of your body need to hold themselves up. No matter how much you relax, the ground beneath rises up to hold you.

Step 3: Focus the relaxation on your hands. The palms seem to expand as they let go of their tension. Feel your fingers soften. There is no effort in your hands, no work for them to do. They are completely open and receptive.

Step 4: Become aware of the places your hands are connected to the "trouble spot" on your body. Give yourself a few breaths to notice the contact points. You don't have to do anything with it; just witness the connection between hands and body.

Step 5: From this relaxed, perceptive state, ask your body if it is willing to communicate with your hands. The answer will not likely come as a "Yes/No" but you will perceive some sense of an answer. It may be as subtle as a willingness or reluctance. If you perceive willingness, proceed to step 6. If you perceive reluctance, enquire, "What stands in the way of you wanting to share?" Respect any feelings, images, or random input to stand as the answer and proceed to step 8.

Step 6: If your body offered a positive sense, or willingness, ask the specific area beneath your hands to share more about its discomfort. You may imagine that your hands themselves are posing the question, with a warm, caring, open energy. Stay receptive to all thoughts, images, and feelings as forms of response from your body. You may ask follow-up questions and remain curious for as long as you can hold the connection with your body and it is responsive to your curiosity. When it seems the dialogue is drawing to a close, ask your body how it wishes to externalize the discomfort.

Step 7: Select an expressive modality that aligned with the kind of answer you received. For example, your body may have clearly let you know it wished to work in color and form, or melody and rhythm. If your body fed you an image, you may draw or paint it. If you felt something, you may dance or create a textile or sculptural work. If it gave you a memory, you might record a short film or write a descriptive paragraph. Do not think about it too much—let your body determine how it wishes to further express its held-in pain.

Step 8: Express from your visceral sense. Do your best to stay connected to your body throughout this process and let it use your hands (or whatever you are creating with) as its conduit. Allow your body to share its truth by unifying your mind with the process: not thinking about, analyzing, or planning what is happening; instead, letting a truth spill out of you, even if it doesn't make sense or look pretty. You may repeat this exercise a number of times with the same area of the body or different areas in order to attune to what is happening within you and unite your body, senses, and mind.

The previous exercise helps tap you into your expressive capabilities beyond your thinking self. The later chapters in this section teach you to harness that thinking mind for the purpose of creation; however, many brilliant expressions can arise when we remove the mental processes from the equation. The following exercise elaborates the nonverbal creative skill and gives you an opportunity to create and express from a purer truth, beyond the limits of language.

Exercise: Connect to Nonverbal Wisdom

Even though it can be tricky to turn off the thinking mind, nay-sayers, and internal analysis, this practice gives you the chance to do all of that. Return to this exercise time and again to free yourself.

Step 1: Commit to not listening to your mind. No "Where should I draw this object? … What am I trying to convey? … Is this graceful enough? …" This exercise is directing you to a pure experience through the body, beyond the thinking mind.

Step 2: Select a nonverbal modality such as visual art, dance, or music. Place your dominant hand in the small of your back and allow your nondominant hand to play in the realm you have selected. If you are moving, be sure to lead with the nondominant side of your body. Do your best to stay connected to how you feel throughout the process.

Step 3: As you continue to create from this nondominant and hopefully nonverbal space, you may notice your mind trying to "help" by offering suggestions, feedback, insights, and other commentary. You may not be able to stop it from doing so; however, you do not need to listen to it. Disregard the words in your mind and continue creating from your body sense. You may be surprised by what is stored beyond the realm of language within you.

Any time you notice your thoughts or programming getting in the way of your creative process, let your nonverbal wisdom shine through. A simple path to quelling the nay-saying thinking mind is to lead creation from your nondominant hand.

Pranayama

Breathing, the fourth limb of the eightfold path, is about the vital force that is carried on the breath (*prana*). By focusing on, controlling, or elongating the inhales (*puraka*), exhales (*rechaka*), and pauses between each (*kumbhaka* and *sunyaka*), we gain mastery over our own vital force. The breath is the bridge between mind and body. When you breathe deeply, your nervous system responds parasympathetically—in other words, you relax. Besides, a relaxed nervous system translates through the emotions and mind, soothing you and slowing your thoughts. In this relaxed state, we are better able to shift perspectives, gain insights, and receive creative inspiration. Although it is beyond the scope of this book, I highly recommend you seek out research on the relationship between relaxation and mental/emotional processes. For now, you can take my word for it. Feel welcome to practice the following exercise, or variation thereof, before settling into any creative endeavor.

Exercise: Breath Practice for Inspiration & Stillness

This practice is simple and powerful in its ability to clear the mind and set the stage for creation. Practice it anytime you feel dull, closed, or uninspired.

Step 1: Come into a comfortable position, sitting or lying down. Without trying to change anything, notice your breath. Does it flow smoothly or stutter? Is it deep? Can you feel it in the front and back of your body? Accept how it is moving in this moment, without trying to change it. If you practice this exercise regularly, you will come to realize how the movement of the breath reflects various internal states.

Step 2: Begin to focus on the inhale and the pause between it and the exhale. Gradually elaborate that pause.

Step 3: Focus on the stillness that rests between the breath phases. As you retain the inhale (*kumbhaka*), notice a sense of fullness. You may connect with an intention and imagine yourself breathing in that quality, holding and distributing its energy as you retain your breath. Remember that what we focus on in practice becomes stronger within us.

This energizing breathing practice elaborates your connection to stillness, improves cognition and concentration, and stretches you from the inside. Perhaps it also helps invigorate you and creates space for fertile ideas.

Calling the Senses to Their Source

The next step on the *Raja* Path is "Sense Mastery" (*pratyahara*). Since our sense organs only offer us limited perception, it is best not to put too much stock in them. On the other hand, as creatives, what we see, hear, and feel is important to our process and how we are able to express ourselves. The yogis teach that the senses have the power to disrupt the mind if we believe them too deeply.

Pratyahara is the process of calling the senses back to their source and drawing them into our consciousness, the way a turtle draws its limbs and head into its shell. By stilling the senses, we know a deeper stillness in the mind. The true Self shines through that mental stillness, as it is often our busy thoughts and fleeting emotions that stand between us and authentic inner connection. The following practice helps quiet sensory overload. (For more practices for the senses, see chapter 10.)

Exercise: Refining Your Senses

This practice helps harness your sensory power by exploring creative media through various sensory foci. It might be best to do a different step each day for five days. Enjoy the process below and use it as a springboard to your own sense-training practices. Be creative in everyday life as you experiment with how your senses, and by extension your mind, interact with the world around you.

Step 1: Listen to one instrument in a song. Let the sounds of all the other instruments simply wash over you as you continually return your attention to the instrument of choice. When that instrument is not playing, enjoy its silence.

Step 2: Gaze at a beautiful scene. Allow your eyes to take in the entire view at once, rather than focusing on any specific thing in the scene. Feel a sense of broadening and relaxation in your eyes, your mind, and your perceptions. If something specific catches your attention, just zoom back out so you are perceiving the whole scene again.

Step 3: Go somewhere far outside the city, burn incense, hold a fragrant flower/herb, or diffuse essential oils. Sit in a relaxed, upright position, close your eyes, and focus on the nasal passage and beyond. Notice, but do not get attached to, the movements of the mind. Allow the aroma to fill your nostrils.

Step 4: Set aside a half hour to spread lotion over your hands, feet, limbs, torso, neck, and face. Take your time with the motion of rubbing it in, using different pressures and qualities of strokes. Be present with the sensory information that your body sends as the touch moves through different qualities and areas. You may also experiment with touching different textures in your home, such as steel, wood, silk, cotton, water, pets, stucco, etc.

Step 5: Set a small morsel of food in front of you. Ideally this is three to five wholesome ingredients in a pretty form. Eat it very slowly, beginning with licking it or putting it in your mouth and rolling it around. Wait before you chomp into the food, allowing yourself contact with the essence of its flavors and how they combine. Chew slowly as you indulge in this morsel. Notice the nuances of flavors that come through, how they change over time, along with how it seems to taste different on different parts of your tongue.

Use a step from this exercise anytime you feel that the busyness and overstimulation of the world is pushing too hard against you.

By learning to master your sensory input, rather than being heavily influenced by external stimuli or even your own thoughts and emotions, you clear your mind and set the stage for upliftedness and pure creative expression. The next step of the eightfold path arises naturally from *pratyahara*.

Mental Focus

When we focus the senses inward instead of letting them lead the mind into the outer world, we become more self-determined and focused. This mental strength is the next limb of the eightfold path: *dharana*, or concentration. Concentration is simply a commitment to set the mind on one idea.

The nature of the mind is to jump around very quickly; like a curious puppy, it wanders here and there exploring all kinds of things. However, just like a puppy, we can train the mind to "stay." In order to practice *dharana*, set your focus on one thing, such as the task at hand, your breath, or an uplifting word or phrase, and every time it wanders away, bring it back to the point of concentration. After a few days or weeks of practicing focus, your mind will become much stronger and better trained. The next step on the eightfold path arises naturally from this.

Meditation

Contrary to popular culture's verbiage, the seventh step of meditation (*dhyana*) is not something we "do." It is a state. When we calmly focus the mind for a time (step 6, *dharana*), consciousness shifts. Similar to how we move from waking to sleep, so concentration shifts to meditation. In meditation our brain waves and physiology alter. This relaxed state of heightened perception is observable when we are caught up in our art. Many of the exercises in this book may elicit a meditative state if you focus on them completely. If you wish to understand your meditation type and establish a daily practice, check out *Meditation for Your Life* by Robert Butera.

Since you likely don't have the technology to prove when you have shifted state, let a sense of general well-being be your benchmark. If you get so swept up in something you lose track of time, that is another simple measure that you likely shifted consciousness. Meditation (*dhyana*) is also notable in the everyday reduction of stress and ability to view most situations from a higher, more peaceful, or more creative perspective.

Superconsciousness

As the brain establishes an open pathway to meditative consciousness, it gradually deepens its spiritual interaction with life. In time, prolonged interaction with states of meditation (*dhyana*) lead to the superconscious state of *samadhi*, or enlightenment, our final step in the eightfold path. Remember that there are many levels of enlightenment; an entire chapter of the *Yoga Sutras* is dedicated to this state. Simply realizing there is such a thing as enlightenment makes you a part of it. The suggestion is to not get too caught up in whether you are or aren't experiencing *samadhi*. Acknowledge the moments when you feel peaceful, connected, and completely well. Spend more time doing things that cultivate that flavor and associate with others who are also interested in feeling that way more often. Do good works in the world: see a need—meet the need. These are the everyday ways of practicing enlightened living. We discuss this more in chapter 14.

When we restrain harm (*yama*), cultivate purity (*niyama*), move in healthy ways and relax ourselves (*asana*), breathe well (*pranayama*), don't believe everything our senses tell us (*pratyahara*), and still the mind (*dharana*), then we shift consciousness (*dhyana*). When we live in that shifted consciousness, we're living from the soul or creative Self. Then we are living in *samadhi,* the superconscious state. Those are the eight steps of *Raja* Yoga that align us with who we truly are. That's the path of the system. The next chapter discusses the path of the heart, *Bhakti.*

Chapter 8
From the Heart

THE PATH THIS CHAPTER focuses on is *Bhakti,* or the devotional path. Folks who follow the *Bhakti* Path tend to be heart-centered: caring, emotional, and sensitive. They tend to be attuned to their own feelings and those of others. Although it isn't always the case, *Bhakti* Yogis tend to be empaths—perceiving others' emotions almost as their own— and body-based. People on the *Bhakti* Path create because they *love it.* Because of this tender level of perception, many artists follow this path to at least some degree. From an enlightenment perspective, people on the path of devotion do well to dedicate themselves to a higher power or purpose, placing their efforts in the hands of love and feeling supported by the spiritual world. In this way, emotions become a tool to connection with the creative Self.

Emotionally or body-based perceivers, especially those who are more sensitive to others' emotions, have a tendency to become overwrought. Our society tends to devalue the information and intuitive reasoning that can come through our emotional sense. This leads to problems processing through emotions and their inherent messages. Instead, we are inclined to partially or completely stifle our emotions until we become addicts or depressives, or we explode. This chapter helps you choose a healthier, unitive path. Learn to use your emotional sensibilities to inspire your creative work and connect to the inner creator. Read on to practice soothing your emotions, connecting to their source and to imagination, and expressing them. The following exercise gets you started with a yoga practice to integrate and balance emotions.

 Exercise: Feeling Soothed Relaxation

This is a gentle, self-loving practice. Although it may bring up worries at first, as you practice it over time your nervous system will associate it with a chance to let those concerns go and feel more deeply soothed and relaxed.

Step 1: Settle in a comfortable place and position. You can choose a traditional relaxation posture like Corpse Pose on your back or curling up in Child's Pose, but any position that lets you feel safe and relaxed will do. You may choose to cover yourself with a blanket and tuck it in close around you. For additional nervous system comfort, add the gentle weight of some cushions over your thighs, abdomen, and chest. Become present through a mindfulness check of body, breath, thoughts, feelings, and overall sense of connection to who you really are.

Step 2: Begin to pay attention to the moment you are in. Notice how good it feels to rest: you don't have to serve anyone, there is no other task in front of you, even your muscles don't have to put forth effort right now. All you have to do is be as you are. That's okay.

Step 3: As you allow yourself to let down, you may notice unprocessed emotions, situations, or lists crop up in your mind. That's a sign of the mind unwinding its stresses. Similarly, your feelings may appear more complex, flurried, or agitated. Yuck, step 3 is uncomfortable … just keep breathing while you feel the floor and the pillows holding you. Usually the discomfort passes and you discover an even deeper layer of relaxation and ease.

Turn to this exercise any time you need to let go of a busy day, intense feelings, or a sense of being overwhelmed. It helps you process without playing into the stresses and teaches the nervous system to stay relaxed, even when the mind becomes busy or confused.

The Creative Child

When we go home to the heart, we often move through many layers of pain before we land back in the sweetness that is or was our original state in this life. I suggest to you that is one of our greatest obstacles in being creative people: in order to truly express ourselves, we must somehow be connected to that sweet, tender presence. For most of us, that place is too tender to let go unguarded and still function in this world. I say tender because there is that sense of easily bruising. When we put ourselves out there creatively, it's a great tenderness.

The beauty of *Bhakti*, the path of the heart, is that we are devoting ourselves to the higher Self first. If you are a religious person, this tenderness rests in God's hands. If you believe in the grand design, then remember that because we are a creation on this planet (no matter what created us), we are of Creation; ergo, we are creative. When we create, whether we are tender or not, we are aligned with the divine Self. In this way, the divine Self and the inner child both have a mystical quality to them.

As we remain tender and connect to the inner child and divine Self, the *Bhakti* Path may require the most courage of all the paths. It may also be the path that best helps us as creators because children—even inner children of adults—are so imaginative.

How connected do you feel to that younger, inventive self? It is the part of us that is free, playful, and trusting. Do you remember feeling open, limitless, and curious about all that may be possible? When we are present in life and open to the opportunity of any given moment, we create best. The trick is that because the inner child self winds up being the sweetest and tenderest part of our adult selves, it can be painful to get or stay in touch with that inner aspect. It can be easy for the adult self to be enlightened—once we are free from the pain of our past. When we experience the *klesas* discussed in part 1 of this book, we are battling with old emotional impressions and *karmas*. Triggers, or people/stimuli/situations that bring strong emotional reactions, are cues about unresolved pain. The following exercise has you reflect upon the childhood experiences that may be blocking your connection to freedom, imagination, and possibility. Repeat the following exercise as often as you like to discern the truth about the roots of your emotional reactions.

Exercise: Excavating the Roots of Emotionally Charged Events

This exercise gives you the opportunity to investigate the source of some of your triggers. If you have a history of abuse or trauma, it may be wise not to attempt this on your own. Bring the exercise into therapy and investigate your emotions with your counselor. If you play with this on your own and find yourself overwhelmed, please breathe slowly and contact a local crisis line to receive support. Conversely, you may enjoy the process of investigating all the emotionally charged events that occur in your everyday life. As you come to understand the source of those charges, it is as if you are diffusing the emotional time bomb within.

Step 1: Think of recent time you experienced heightened emotion. Allow the situation and emotion to reoccur and witness it. Stay connected to that observant, calm part of yourself as you call the emotion in. Notice how the emotion/situation impacts what is going on in your body. What happens to your muscles, back, abdomen, and face? Are there specific parts of your body that seem to react more than others? How is your breathing? What thoughts arise? Notice the story you tell yourself about this emotion and situation.

Step 2: Remain connected to your calm witness self as well as your body and breath. Continue relaxing, even though the emotion is heightened. Ask yourself, *When was the first time I remember feeling this way?* and allow whatever happens within you to happen. You may remember a few weeks ago when a similar situation arose or a long time ago when something impactful happened. Repeat your observation process from step 1 to explore the earlier exposure to this emotion as deeply as you can. Remain connected to your calm witness as you observe.

Step 3: When you have identified and observed the first time you remember feeling this way, express the emotion with movement and sound. You might flail, dance, collapse, clap, roll around on the floor, or all of these things and more! Give sound to the movement as you roar, moan, holler, laugh, hum, etc. Give over to the embodiment of the emotion and the sounds it can make. If it helps, you can put music on.

Step 4: When you feel finished with moving the emotion, rest in a relaxation posture and consciously feel yourself letting go. The Feeling Soothed Relaxation in this chapter is a good practice now.

The yogis call these trigger-reaction patterns *samskara* and the scientists call it neuroplasticity. Both the ancient and modern concepts speak to the idea that once we have established a pathway, we will continue to walk that same cognitive/emotional route time and again. As a conscious creator, you have the ability to choose differently. Now that you are aware of your habit and where it comes from, it is easier to be creative and ask yourself what other options are available.

Imagination & the Creative Child

There are many popular works that can help you connect to your creative essence. At some point, each of these works has you reflect upon your childhood: the pains, programming, interests, and joys that uniquely shaped you. There are a number of reasons why our inner children carry keys to our creative victories. Children are tender, imaginative, and playful. Under the best of circumstances they are not self-conscious. Really young ones don't understand the laws of our physical reality and believe all kinds of uncanny and brilliant things are possible.

You yourself may have had some wild ideas about the way you hoped the world could be. Before I understood that television wasn't spying on characters in their own homes, I thought that animated figures were people in another country. Their faces and houses looked different from ours, just as in my own neighborhood there were folks of varying heights, complexions, and aesthetic tastes. Connect to your own sense of imaginative possibility through the following exercise.

Exercise: Open Your Perceptions to the Magic of Life

Forget everything you think you know about the laws of life and physical reality—it's time to play.

Step 1: Think back to when you were very little and didn't know much about the world. Many people find it hard to connect back that far and that's okay. Even if you don't concretely remember being confused by cars, technology, adult relationships, church, animals, or whatever, open yourself to a sense of the world being very big. If you are really creative, you will finish out this step by crawling around your house for five to ten minutes, or staying very low, as you explore the world from the perspective of a young one.

Step 2: Now that you have connected to that sense of being much smaller than your environment, get specific about what used to confuse you or the strange ideas you may have had about life. If you don't remember them, just let yourself be silly now and think outside of the box. For example, in addition to thinking I was a voyeur into cartoon characters' lives, I also believed that since "God is everywhere" and outer space is so big, we probably lived in God's foot. Maybe you thought that the bathtub drain would swallow you or the animals you saw in clouds could actually come to life. Let your mind wander back and daydream about the weird concepts you explored as a child.

Step 3: Select one of these ideas and paint it with your nondominant hand. If you have tempera paints and a largish brush like you used in preschool, all the better. Notice, as your nondominant hand struggles to convey what your brain imagines, what it is like to be in a body that doesn't have fine motor control yet. This, too, is a remembrance of childhood.

Step 4 (optional): You may use your work from step 3 as inspiration for a truly beautiful and heartfelt adult piece.

Step 5: Now that you have opened your mind to your inner child, remain perceptive to other strange ideas and points of view that may arise in everyday life. Is that birdcall a hidden message? Does your art make more sense upside down? Do fairies live in your garden? What happens if you do everything backward?

May this childlike view of a magical world help you cultivate compassion for your ideas and emotions as they arise, as well as tether you to creative inspiration...and open your perceptions to the magic of life!

" … As though Everything Is a Miracle … "

If we look at the world with the eyes of a tender-hearted child or imaginative creator, then we perceive those nuances of how the world itself is fit together. Einstein had the idea of seeking meaning in every experience. If everything is a miracle, then we have a continual compass needle pointing in the direction of joy and purity. People on the *Bhakti* Path, who are prone to emotional sensitivity and tender reactions, also have a great capacity for joy. This is the flip side of an open heart. The gift yoga therapy brings you is a guide for elevating beyond everyday, changeable emotions and connecting to a steady, pervasive truth. Joy is a virtue. It is a sustained, soulful quality. As one on the *Bhakti* Path, you are predisposed for a greater capacity for joy because you are already living from a heart-centered perspective. Attuning to—or searching for—continual miracles can anchor you in a joyful sense of the everyday. The following exercise begins to cultivate the skill of perceiving miracles.

Exercise: Discover Signposts That You Are On the Creative Path

One of the ways to open your *bhakti* heart and truly fall in love with life is to perceive the miracles all around you. If you are the creator of your life then there must be some kind of signpost or way of marking the true path. Let's play with that idea:

Step 1: Have an intention. Know what you are creating. This is important in the broad sense and you have been setting intentions throughout this book. Now, refine one of those intentions to something very specific. What do you need or want from today? In time, you can create more amazing things; for now, pick something small. An event you could dismiss as coincidence is easier for your nay-sayers to deal with until they grow accustomed to your creative prowess. Some examples might be to cheer someone up, have your big project finish smoothly, find change on the sidewalk, or encounter a cute animal. Note that it is wise to set intentions that benefit more people than just yourself.

Step 2: Look at life with the eyes of a creator. Intend to create magic. Although you created a specific intention in step 1, remember that there may be a larger force at play (one with a sense of humor, I might add!) and you are actually cocreating miracles with this benevolent force. Hold your intention with you but stay open to other ways the world may offer you joy, opportunity, and ease.

Step 3: At the end of the day, record all the happy coincidences and moments of joy that you experienced.

Step 4: Repeat this process every day for a determined period (I recommend a moon cycle: four weeks). Notice that the coincidences amplify and you grow more adept at manifesting your pure intention.

As you establish a daily practice of observing, cooperating with, and even cultivating wonder in life, you grow closer to your innocence and true creative vision. Any pure thing we practice with dedication bolsters our hearts and connects us to something deeper within ourselves.

Devotion & the *Bhakti* Path

As we deepen our yoga, artistic, or other spiritual practice, *bhaktas'* hearts continue to strengthen and open. In the depth of our soulful hearts is a deep devotion to our practice: we love it. And practice loves us in return. We do not practice in order to receive rewards; however, the rewards are implicit: when we pray or meditate, our physiology sets to a more healthful state (for ourselves *and* others). When we create, we free our expression and end up with a personal reflection more telling than any mirror; when we attend a place of worship—be it temple, band hall, or dance studio—our community embraces and sees us. This cycle of devotional practice/spiritual rewards can lead us to a truly loving, joyful, and enlightened place. Practice both emboldens and uplifts us. The following exercise lets you explore that.

Exercise: Staying Connected to Devoted Practices: The Heartfelt Gift to Yourself

When we understand how and why we do something, it is easier to maintain and create similar habits and behaviors. This exercise inspires your confidence and builds heartfelt devotion.

Step 1: Identify a nourishing habit you have. This could be nightly walks, morning meditation, a gratitude journal … anything that you perform on a regular basis that makes you feel calm or healthy.

Step 2: Acknowledge how you were able to form that habit. Did you just start up one day and stick with it continually or was it a process? If it was a process, how did you keep it up when you were reluctant or busy?

Step 3: When you didn't want to but performed the habit anyway, *why* did you? How did it feel after you pushed through and made it happen? Call upon your creative resources to express that feeling: move, write, whistle, etc.

A devoted practice feeds us twice: once through the healthy practice itself and a second time through the esteem of knowing we can stick to something and deserve to care for ourselves. As a creative person on a heart-centered path, do your best to hold the importance of self-love and self-nurturance in mind. These comforting, healthful habits become routines that feed but are not held prisoner by intense emotions. Such routines are a bridge to the creative Self. The next exercise can help you move beyond fear so that you may continue to take such actions.

Exercise: Yoga Posture Practice: I'm No Cowardly Lion: Using Lion Pose to Transform Fears

The creative path requires strength. Although emotionally driven people are accused of being too sensitive, it actually takes great courage to feel emotions and live a devotional life. Use this exercise to identify and stay connected to your lionheartedness.

Step 1: Identify an emotion or a situation that scares you. (Remember, courage doesn't mean not afraid. If we weren't afraid, we wouldn't *need* the courage.)

Step 2: Shape your body into a representation of that fear. This could be standing, seated, or lying down, in motion or still. There is no right or wrong; simply trust your body to make a shape. Notice how this shape affects your musculature, breath, thoughts, and emotions. How creative do you feel right now? Where are your senses of freedom, trust, and joy? While you hold this shape, how is the feeling/situation you're afraid of behaving or moving around your body (inside or outside)?

Step 3: Imagine putting that feeling/situation in a cage in front of you. This is a magical cage that holds it until you say "Release." Examine what is in the cage. Does it have a shape, color, movement pattern, face, or voice? What, if anything, does it want from or for you? Draw it, paint it, or collage a representation of its energy.

Step 4: Have a sip of water. Sit on your heels, cross-legged, or on a chair with feet on the floor. Keep your back straight and your fingers splayed over your knees, palms down. Take a deep breath in, widen your fierce eyes, open your mouth fully, stick your tongue toward your chin, and *roar!* Press the air right from the belly with the throat open and relaxed so it does not strain. Your roar may be silent, "*Ahhh,*" "*RAAAAAAR,*" or whatever else feels natural. (I know, it feels weird. Keep practicing—it'll get natural. I promise.) This is *Simhasana*, Lion's Pose.

Step 5: Stand up with legs hip-width apart, feet flat on the floor, knees slightly bent. Spread your palms on your knees or thighs and repeat the entire pose. Be sure to consciously direct your roar at the thing in the cage and do not strain your vocal apparatus. Allow the roar to be open and expressive, supported by the diaphragm.

Step 6: Re-examine what is in the cage. How does it move or hold its "body"? If it has eyes, look into them. What does it seem to want from or for you? On a fresh page, draw, paint, or collage its energy.

Step 7: Tell the feeling/situation what you want it to know. Do your best to affirm yourself via this exchange. Notice the response from the creature in the cage. Draw, paint, collage, or write your self-affirming message and post in a place you will see it often.

Step 8 (optional): If your relationship with the caged creature is transformed, it may now be a close ally. Did it teach you about yourself and your capacity for courage? Can you come to a healthy agreement with it? If so, set it free. In this way, you are freeing an aspect of your creative Self, as well.

Sometimes our emotions are so strong they spin a believable story. This exercise gave you the chance to perceive and create a different point of view. It takes courage to move beyond our intense emotions and fears.

The *Bhakti* Path harnesses the power of our emotions to cultivate a life of freedom, imagination, devotion, and joy. Although it sometimes takes courage to face what triggers our feelings, all of it deserves expression and may be the source of beautiful creations. The next chapter takes you from the realm of feelings into an intellectual approach as you create from a sense of wisdom on the *Jnana* Path.

Chapter 9
Think It Through

THE NEXT PATH IS for those who prefer to *study it*. *Jnana* (pronounced with a hard "g," GHEE-ahn-ah) means wisdom or knowledge and is a path for the thinker. Scientists, mathematicians, engineers, and folks who tend to be logical may prefer the *Jnana* Path. What may be called "left-brained" types can also bring a great deal of power to what is typically thought of as the "right-brained" realm of creativity. On the *Jnana* Path, people are thinking about enlightenment—or in this case creativity—and educating themselves about it, following recommendations and ideas that arise from their studies.

By approaching a creative project with the curiosity of a scientist, many ideas, theories, and techniques can inspire beautiful works of art and opportunities for personal expression. Through studying personal interests and taking an objective, scientific approach to creativity, you can follow your intellectual curiosity and access your creative Self.

Pursuing Interests

As we have already discussed, what we create need not be a traditional artistic piece, such as a novel or painting, but may also be an invention, theorem, or alternative application. Any time we develop an idea, we are creating. Ingenuity can arise from pursuing or investigating others' ideas and approaches.

It is possible to gain creative inspiration from any field of study that interests you, be it quantum physics, history, or mechanical engineering. The great artist Leonardo DaVinci is a great example of a creator on the path of *jnana*. He studied and acquired wisdom regarding the relationship between the human form—and indeed many aspects of nature—and geometry. His enquiry into flight was a precursor to modern flying machines. His investigations into the science of the natural world may be some of what continues to make his paintings so touching to this day. Observe yourself and notice what academic topics get you excited. This enthusiasm is a key gateway to your creative soul.

Another way to access inspiration on the *Jnana* Path is by studying other creators in your field. If you are an inventor, you may be interested in how Isaac Newton, Thomas Edison, or Alexander Graham Bell lived. As a portraitist, you may study the beliefs and efforts of Mendelson Joe or Arcimboldo. Actors would do well to watch some James Lipton episodes and review acclaimed performances. Be inquisitive about how they created, what and why, together with the nature of their cadence, brush-strokes, or gestures and how they related colors, emphasis, or themes.

An intellectual or academic awareness of others' processes and styles supports your own development. Through the acquisition of knowledge, you also gain wisdom about yourself and your craft. Our creative studies teach us about who we are and steer us away from who we are not. Investigation refines our efforts and processes.

Exercise: Studying Your Craft

This exercise directs you in a method of applying knowledge to your own creative process. While some folks may feel that an intellectual approach is antithetical to a creative work, one on the *Jnana* Path feels free to create once the research is complete. This studious structure offers inspiration by way of your own wisdom and intellectual preparedness.

Step 1: Take one or two minutes to brainstorm on a piece of paper as many art forms you can think of that pique your curiosity.

Step 2: Circle the three modalities that interest you most at this time. For each of these, brainstorm a few ways you could learn more about each one. For example, you could learn about film by studying various directors, writers, or actors or by reviewing the career of a single director, writer, or actor. You could learn more about tattoos by visiting local shops to view their portfolios or interview the artists. You could research techniques and theories, peruse magazines, take a class, or watch a documentary.

Step 3: Pick the one modality and research method that is most appealing to you right now. If you wish, you can tuck away this list and revisit it anytime your creative well is running dry.

Step 4: After completing some research—an hour is sufficient—set a timer for twenty minutes and apply what you have learned. Create something using the information you just gathered, an idea that occurred to you during your studies, or by practicing a technique you discovered. (The timer helps limit any overthinking or judgment that may occur, which are a couple of challenges the intellectual may face.)

Challenges on the *Jnana* Path

Jnanis are thinkers. This chapter applies your intellectual prowess to your creative life and helps you use it as motivation. The flip side of a thinking creator is "overthinking." One of the easiest ways any of us limits our inventiveness is by getting in our own way, and the thought-processes of judgment and analysis can be paralyzing. It is important, especially for one on the *Jnana* Path, to take time to plan and strategize; however, too much thinking, or thinking that interrupts action, is counterproductive.

The suggestion is for you to notice the content of your thoughts. The following exercise gives you a concrete tool to transcend your thinking mind. From that place of discernment, you can filter through your thoughts and use your intellectual prowess to better yourself and your creative outcomes.

Exercise: Steering the Mind: Practicing Discernment through Mindfulness & Movement

Ancient yoga theory in the *Upanishads* teaches us that there are layers of thinking that happen within us. There is the mind, which we might consider the busy passing thoughts, everyday ramblings, and emotional turns within us. Then there is the intellect, which we can think of as longer-held, more entrenched beliefs and steadfast thought patterns. When used effectively, the intellect also offers discernment, steering the mind in the direction we wish to follow.

Step 1: Sit or, if you don't have balance issues, stand comfortably in a symmetrical posture. Close your eyes. Notice the contents of your mind. What thoughts are there? What emotions do you notice? Your thoughts might seem to speed up when you try this, and your feelings could press in a little too close. It's okay; that's how the mind unwinds sometimes.

Step 2: Remain aware of your thoughts and feelings, but put more focus to your breath. Notice what parts of your abdomen, chest, sides, and back are moving as you inhale and exhale.

Step 3: Open your eyes, breathe in, and stretch your arms overhead. If you were sitting, stand up now. Lean yourself a little to one side and then the other as you breathe deeply, in your own form of gentle side bends. Straighten up, then lift your chest and chin into a slight back bend, creating space through the front of the body as you lengthen your abdomen, chest, and throat slightly forward and upward. Next, roll forward, letting your head and arms hang in a forward fold, then firm your belly and roll back up to standing. Twist your upper body from side to side, rotating at the waistline, ribs, chest, shoulders, and head. Enjoy great big, deep breaths all the while.

Step 4: Return to your original position and repeat step 1. Did you notice a difference this time? Were your thoughts slower and more recognizable after the movements? We would anticipate this, as gentle movements help process emotional refuse via the autonomic nervous system and set us back into a parasympathetic, or more relaxed, physiological state. It can take some practice for the body to offer up that response, however. Study yourself and notice what kinds of movements help you feel more relaxed.

Step 5: Continue watching your thoughts and feelings ... then picture a bird. Picture a tree. Imagine a little tune. How did you do that? Is there a part of you that can actually tell your mind what to think?!

Step 6: Consider a motto, prayer, or credo that is important to you at this time. Whenever you notice yourself becoming too judgmental, direct your thoughts back to this deeper intention and let it direct your activities. Remember that you are the master of your mind and have the power to choose your thoughts and mental experiences.

Whenever we find ourselves stuck in thinking rather than action, it helps to just acknowledge that it has happened. Being mindful of and redirecting our thoughts are the best ways to get out of our heads and back into action. The rest of this chapter offers a scientific model, via the metaphor of the butterfly, to support you in continuing your creative efforts, especially when you get bogged down in judgment or lose faith in how the project will turn out.

Think of a Butterfly

It is beneficial to apply intellectual understanding to our inventive efforts. Considering the life cycle of a butterfly helps inform the creative process itself. Just as a butterfly moves through distinct phases on its journey to perfection, so your creation—and indeed your inner world—passes through phases on the journey of expression. The *Jnana* Path supports you in understanding how and why to stick with a project, even when it gets tough. Another piece of wisdom on this path may inform when it is time to let something go or label it complete. Another advantage is to begin knowing that the end already exists; it is just a matter of passing through the phases to see it realized. Note how alike the process of creation and the process of life are in the following sections.

Exercise: Yoga Posture Practice: Expressing the Creative Process through the Body

This yoga pose practice takes you through the butterfly process. Imagine yourself embodying each stage and notice the differences in energy, motivation, safety, and inspiration.

Step 1: Use your body to create the shape of an egg. You may choose a Child's Pose (*Balasana*), curled up on the floor with your seat toward your heels and your forehead on the ground or stacked fists, or you may curl up in a ball on your back, with your knees toward your chest (*Apanasana*). Imagine yourself protected in the dark, quiet space of creation. Feel the smallness of your physical self and the vastness of your potential. Rest as long as you need to in the shelter of the egg.

Step 2: When you are ready to emerge, express an unfolding. Stay connected to your body as you expand and sprout outward. Bring yourself onto your abdomen and reach your arms overhead. Very gently, begin to curve your entire spine so that your arms and legs lift off the ground. Direct your eyes to the floor and feel the strength in your back. This is a version of Locust Pose (*Shalabhasana*).

Step 3: Continue growing, letting yourself rise up to seated or standing, perhaps walking around the room. Explore your environment as if it were all brand new, as if you were a new life form on this planet. You may think of this as the larva stage.

Step 4: Use circles to express movement. You may walk in circles or spin yourself like a slow top carefully around the room. Every so often pause and create a standing twisted posture (*Kati Chakrasana*) by holding the hips and legs still while revolving the upper body around in a simple standing twist. You can also try keeping the upper body still and rotating the feet to face ninety degrees from your torso, so that the twisting action seems to come from the lower body. Experiment with various arm positions, such as reaching out to the sides, overhead, or hugging yourself. Remember to even out the twist on both sides so that you twist to the right and left. Imagine that the spiraling action is like a caterpillar spinning a cocoon.

Step 5: Reach your arms overhead and grow to your full height, just as a caterpillar realizes its own potential during its time in the cocoon. When you are ready, stretch wide in all directions to burst out of the chrysalis.

Step 6: Move in new ways. You may walk sideways instead of forward, using your peripheral vision to guide the action (be safe and aware of your environment all the while). Pause, bring your legs hip-width apart, and raise your arms overhead, hands in line with shoulders. Keep your hips stable and strong as you bend sideways to the left, then to the right, one side then the other, in a version of Half Moon Pose (*Ardha Chandrasana*). Imagine you are a butterfly growing accustomed to your new body. Repeat the lateral walking and the lateral bend a few times.

Step 7: Move however and wherever you wish. Just as the butterfly is free to soar where it wishes, you are free: a light, colorful creature of earth and sky.

Now that you have played with growing the way a butterfly grows, we will look at how your creative process moves through phases like a butterfly. This supports your scientific view of your inventive life.

The Egg

As in creating life, so in creating art: life starts with a seed or an egg, creations start with ideas. Within the seed lies the potential. Every mighty oak with all its beautiful colored leaves started off the little nut of an acorn. Our ideas are these seeds within us, or the egg that is coded with all the potential it needs to realize its eventual perfection. An acorn does not look like an oak; an egg does not look like a butterfly; a pile of metal does not look like a shiny, rebuilt engine. However, within the beginning lies the end. Everything needed to complete a venture—be it life or a single expressive piece—is already within the idea. When you look at an acorn you see a mere seed not a great tree; an insect egg is not a beautiful butterfly; a blank page is not a play. Even though you can't yet see it, when you have an idea, everything you need to express that touching truth is encoded within it.

The Larva

From the egg comes the larva: the wee crawling caterpillar that shuffles from plant to plant. It finds a choice leaf and stays there for a couple of days, munching away. The caterpillar doesn't know its own potential yet. This may be like you when you are outlining your essay, practicing scales, or sketching your painting. There is not the sense of what your efforts could really turn into. Remember, the end was already encoded in the idea. Believe that you are on the cusp of brilliance at all times, you just cannot see it from the proximal perspective of the caterpillar.

The caterpillar's complete view of the world is hunkered down, right up close to things. It is unable to rise above its own scrutiny and see the big picture. When we think about the locomotive pattern of the cater-pillar, we understand that it cannot go just anywhere; its sticky feet and short, shuffling legs can only carry it so far. The caterpillar is able to investigate the world at close range while its main mission is nourish-ment. Although it may not understand what is to come, the impulse to fatten up and get ready is a strong one.

That is like us beginning to grind out a project. Once you hatch the idea you have to get started. You gather the materials that you need, organize the ideas, and dive in. This is an indulgent phase. It feels so good to get going on a new idea! The creation comes easily; we are full of new life and vigor. Just as the caterpillar sheds its skin many times, so you may go through many forms of your idea as you shape it. There is a great deal of energy at the beginning of the creative process. Surf this wave as long as you can, my friend, because you are going to need all the nourishment you can get in the phase that comes next.

Exercise: How to Nourish Your Creative Self

There are many ways to nourish ourselves. Proper nutrition, be it physical, emotional, mental, or spiritual, makes us resilient enough to go through the more challenging aspects of creation. Use this practice to bolster yourself and stay strong.

Step 1: List the healthy things you do to take care of your-self when you are working on a big project. Do you take deep breaths and stretching breaks, call your friends, go for a walk, keep music playing...?

Step 2: List the not-so-healthy things you do to cope with the stress when you are in the middle of a project. Do you drink, smoke, pick fights, procrastinate...?

Step 3: Look at both lists. Draw happy shapes around the habits that you welcome in your life or feel proud that you engage in. Draw boxes around the habits that make you feel uncomfortable, remorseful, or ashamed.

Step 4: On a new sheet of paper, draw two columns and list the pleasing strategies in one and the displeasing ones in the other. Be the sleuth and investigate what is similar and different about the items in both columns. In other words, how is picking fights similar to calling your friends? How is smoking like deep breathing? How is going for a walk like drinking alcohol? How are they different?

Step 5: Scientists include a "therefore" in their study write-ups. What conclusion can you draw about what you need to nourish yourself while working on a project?

    a. Often, our unhealthy habits give clues to what is missing in our lives. Once we are aware of those missing pieces, we can find healthy ways to give them to ourselves.

    b. We can build on healthy habits, letting the feel-good nature of self-care blossom in our everyday lives. For most of us, what truly helps us cope are often small things like looking out the window or at a pleasing image in our workspace.

Step 6: Considering the similar threads that ran through your coping strategies, take one small action right now to incorporate more of that nourishment into your everyday life. This may be adding time for a walk, bath, nap, or phone call into your schedule, putting your favorite fruit on the grocery list, or creating a motivational playlist.

The Cocoon

Once the caterpillar has obtained enough mass, it sheds a final layer of skin and reveals its chrysalis. It is time to weave the pupa and enter the cocoon, where metamorphosis takes place. Your creative work also goes through a painful transformation and remembering the life of the butterfly can help keep you motivated during those tougher times in the process.

When I was in graduate school studying expressive arts and counseling, my mentor asked me to consider how a caterpillar feels within the cocoon. She was teaching me about the process of personal growth and highlighting the point that therapy is not good times. Breaking through often means breaking down. She spelled it out for me: "It's dark, cramped, wet..." I had never thought of it before—the cocoon might not be such a nice place. "You are becoming a new kind of creature," she continued. "There is no one in the cocoon with you."

It is true! The caterpillar doesn't know it is turning into a beautiful butterfly; it is simply trapped alone in the ache of metamorphosis. It must be uncomfortable! A caterpillar loses half of its mass in the cocoon. It has to be painful sprouting wings. Growth is painful. If you have been in therapy or taken a personal transformation course, you know it can be awful at times. That may be what it is like in the chrysalis. Likewise, that can be what it's like when we create: dark, lonely, unknown, and uncomfortable.

The difference between a metamorphosing bug and a human creator is choice. While we can empathize with the creature in the pupa, unlike them we have the option to walk away from the transformation. If a caterpillar could make that choice, it would mean death. On the other hand, if you decide to drop a project the worst thing that might happen is you miss a chance to know yourself, express something, or enjoy completion. You will survive that (in fact, some projects are best discarded); however, abandonment is not a worthwhile pattern to get into. It is often best to push all the way through a creative quest.

The 80 Percent Rule & Getting It Done

Italian economist Vilfredo Pareto postulated that 80 percent of Italy's wealth was in the hands of 20 percent of the population. As study of the Pareto Principle continued, this 80/20 distribution showed up continually: we hang out with 20 percent of our social circle 80 percent of the time, we wear 20 percent of our clothes 80 percent of the time, we eat 20 percent of our meal repertoire 80 percent of the time. In my world, the same rule applies to tasks. I will readily complete 80 percent of the required work, then feel like I have had enough. I would rather light the whole thing on fire than finish it. I first noticed this 80 percent phenomenon doing dishes: all the plates and the glasses are done; I've wiped down some of the counters. I could change out the dishwater and scrub these three pots or I could just soak them. I'm 80 percent done.

Something happens around 80 percent completion of anything where we just want to quit. We're done. "I'm almost done, so I *am* done." A contributing factor is that the last 20 percent of the project is typically the worst part: editing the screenplay, color correcting the photograph, applying the third coat of varnish to the desk. We can harness that feeling of being "done with" the work and use it to impel completion. What does the butterfly have to do? It does not have the luxury of saying, "Meh, I turned into a butterfly. That was the important part. Now I'm just going to stay here in the cocoon."

Well, that won't do! At that terminal point of the creative project, we almost inevitably consider abandoning it. Maybe the dialogue doesn't work or the lighting in the pictures is not what you want. You could just pack it in but no, help your creation fight out of the cocoon. This last 20 percent is the worst of it and requires a push.

Exercise: Press for Completion

It takes fortitude to push through the last bit of a creative endeavor. This exercise gives you a chance to get stronger and learn more about your barriers as you finish up what for many people is the hardest part.

Step 1: Select a project that is almost finished. This can be something urgent/important or an old work that has been kicking around for awhile. Regard that project as it is: almost but not quite done. Notice all the thoughts, feelings, and analyses that arise. You may jot down or doodle them.

Step 2: Transfer those feelings so that you no longer have a sense of "I am so done with the project" but rather "I am so done in this cocoon. I'm finished with being stuck in here by myself. It hurts!" This cognitive shift displaces the negativity from your wonderful (or even not-so-wonderful) work. It's okay to be irked. Be irked with the cocoon, not your creation.

Step 3: Channel your frustration into completion and allow the full expression of the project you began to see the light of day.

Finish the last 20 percent of your creative projects. Even if you are not thrilled with the end product, the act of 100 percent completion, rather than 80 percent striving, is fulfilling and worthy.

Have you ever watched a butterfly bust out of a cocoon? Is it an easy process? No. It is a grind. The poor butterfly; it is not bad enough it has to reshape its entire body, now it has to crack its way out of this would-be coffin. It's all covered in goo; it is a different shape, a seemingly different creature (even though its DNA is exactly the same as a caterpillar) and it doesn't even know it yet. It must fight its way out of the cocoon and if it can't then that's it, no butterfly. Likewise, when we do not press for completion, we do not know the soaring freedom of a butterfly. We miss out on the new perspectives our finished project may give us.

Exercise: Busting Out of the Cocoon

This exercise empowers you to gain perspective on your work and honor all the efforts that brought you to completion.

Step 1: Identify the difficult endeavor, be it a school/work project, home renovation/cleaning task, or something you loved when it started and now just wish it were done. Go to the workspace where you would complete this task (your desk, where the renovation/cleaning needs to happen, your studio, etc.). Bring some raucous music with you.

Step 2: Play your up-tempo song and move to the music. Be sure to incorporate various levels (high, mid-range, low) with your limbs, torso, and head. Experiment with different facial movements as well. As you move and express, keep the thought of the project with you. Dance out your frustrations, doubts, and resistances. Feel free! Be light! "I can do it! I believe in myself!"

Step 3: Sit down with your project in front of you and close your eyes. Let your spine be long and your torso be erect and strong yet relaxed. Soften your brow, eyes, and jaw. Turn up the corners of your mouth slightly. Witness the flow of your breath and feel your heart slowing.

Step 4: Call to mind an image of yourself working on the project. Maintain the upward curl of the lips and steady, even breathing. Watch yourself performing the required tasks as you would watch your favorite character in a movie montage, hauling materials and mortaring bricks or counting push-ups and running stairs. See yourself moving through all the little jobs you need to do in order to complete the larger project. Your imagination can fill in the victorious theme music.

Step 5: At the end of your montage, see yourself reflecting upon the completed endeavor. Pay close attention to the expression on your face, the gleam in your eyes, the open, confident posture. You did it! As you hold this image, bask in its visceral sense. Allow your entire body-mind complex to light up with the goodness of a job well done.

Step 6: Play your song again or something reminiscent of the theme song you heard during your visualization. Move to the music.

Step 7: This is the fun one: *be* the montage. Get goin'. You can do it!

Step 8: As you move toward completion, notice when you are losing steam, becoming critical, or focusing more on the end goal than the task at hand. Play your song again. You may continue working, as your cells have imprinted the movement and motivation from your recent encounters with this song, or get up and repeat steps 2 through 7.

Step 9: When you have completed the challenging project—made it to your 100 percent point—take time to revel in the victory. When we acknowledge our achievements, there is a neurological pay-off: we get a surge of dopamine (the neurotransmitter "ping" of falling in love, eating chocolate, or getting fifty Facebook "likes" in an hour). Enjoy the healthy biochemical high. Let each success, no matter how small your inner judge tries to scale it, be a triumph worth celebrating. Feel light and free like a soaring butterfly.

When it comes to finishing your creation, the scientist in you thinks, *Just fight through this last bit because once the cocoon is busted I have the freedom of a butterfly. The higher perspective of a butterfly.* Its beauty and sensitivity is a transcendent version of its former self. It can move in any direction now, not limited to wherever it can crawl. The butterfly sees things completely differently. That's us in the creative process. When we are standing on the completed side of our creative endeavor, it mirrors an aspect of our soul back to us.

The finished project tells us something about ourselves that we couldn't see before. Investigating the final work and the process that got us there, as scientists, reveals nuances about our true selves, our patterns, and what we may be going through in life: this is who I was; this is who I am; this is what that was; this is what that means; and so on. By observing processes and outcomes, we come to know our own creative soul via that scientific approach.

When the caterpillar, who is no longer a caterpillar, is done in the chrysalis, it has to fight its way out. This is a metaphor for our own creative process. The closer we are to completion, the harder it may seem to finish the job. Fight for it. Earn your way to freedom. When you are done with the task, consider it a completion of your current level of existence and celebrate the step in your own evolutionary journey.

Exercise: Using Knowledge of the Butterfly to Finish a Tough Project

It is common to get held up before finishing a creation. This might be because of self-doubt, timing, or not knowing what to do next. When nature creates, it trusts the process. Perform this exercise in a similar fashion and see that you can get that project done.

Step 1: Find an old idea that you love but have not been able to get to. Alternatively, you may dredge up a project that is important to you but has stagnated. What is the seed of this project? What is the outcome you envision?

Step 2: Gather nourishment for this idea. Doodle shapes, collect scraps of images, get paint chips for colors, create a soundtrack that goes along with it, list key phrases or snippets of dialogue. You may not actually use these things; however, they help the project grow, just as the caterpillar has long since digested the leaf when it weaves the cocoon.

Step 3: Set a timer for somewhere between twenty and ninety minutes and go at the project. Do not think about it. Do not ruminate. Do whatever you can do to prevent a pause or break in the creative process (keep the pen or brush moving, the music playing, the movement going). You can pare it down later if necessary. Trust that once it has hatched and nourished itself, this idea knows how to grow on its own. The metamorphosing insect is not in the cocoon thinking, *Is this the right place to put this wing? Should I make my leg go here? Is this the right color?* By its very nature, it already knows how to arrive at the perfect outcome. This is the science of creation. Don't mess with it.

Step 4: When the timer rings, you may decide to take a little break. Review your work within a day. Appreciate the little surprises. Celebrate the progress. You deserve it! Show someone else your effort so far and ask for two pieces of supportive feedback.

Step 5: Repeat until rough effort is complete.

This process of approaching the creative task with new tools and trusting the uncontrolled outcomes is valuable. Most butterflies emerge complete and beautiful, even in their imperfections. The same can be true for your works.

Now that you understand the *Jnana* Path is one of inquisitiveness and structure, you can harness that intellectual approach to each of your creative endeavors. From the beginning of a task, you have a vision for the end. You may begin with research, practice, or brainstorming, then build your idea into being. You can be patient with the process, remembering how uncomfortable it must be within the cocoon, all the while understanding that the act of making something has its own determined course. The next chapter broadens your feelings and thoughts into sensory and energetic interactions with the world. You are about to gain inspiration through pleasure and connection on the *Tantra* Path.

Chapter 10
Sensing Creation

THE LAST OF THE five paths we are exploring is the path of *Tantra* Yoga. I know what you are thinking and yes, sex is a creative act; however, true *tantra* is far richer than mere sexual connection. *Tantra* can be thought of as harnessing the subtle senses to transcend our physical awareness. *Tantra* is a path of body-mind health, where attuning ourselves with the energies within and around us provides an abiding perception of unity, inspiration, and clear vision. This subtle, connected sense supports your authentic, passionate self-expression. The creator on the *Tantra* Yoga path *feels it*.

"Feeling" is at the core of much creative work. Intuitive, energetically sensitive people often follow the *Tantra* Path. Through the pleasure of your five senses, self-trust, and intuition you can let your genius shine.

Pleasure

You are probably not surprised that the topic of "pleasure" comes up in the *tantra* chapter. What may surprise you, however, is that the deepest pleasure comes from the realms beyond the physical. Just as you may perceive your creative process as originating from somewhere outside of your consciousness, so the experience of pleasure can be transcendent. We elaborate our idea of pleasure when we think of how pleasurable it is to watch a blank page turn into a story, a canvas become a play of color, or fingers on a piano align with complex harmonies and melodies. There is a richness of pleasure to be derived through the act of connection and creativity.

This creative delight springs from connection with our inner realms. The *Upanishads* teach us that we physical beings contain evermore subtle layers of existence (*koshas*): from the physical body, through the breath-energy (*prana*), the mind/emotions (*manas*), discerning intellect (*vijnana*), to the spiritual realms of bliss (*ananda*). We have easy access to the breath-energy level, which is the plane where our energy meridians (*nadis*) and *chakras* are perceived. A few simple ways to open your perception to the *pranic* realms are to look at the space between tree leaves, shape your hands as if you were holding a ball and "feel" it, or receive an energy treatment such as Reiki. These subtle perceptions can be mentally and emotionally nourishing. The following exercise harmonizes those layers of being and helps tune you in to your subtler perceptions.

 Exercise: Feeling Good through the
Layers of Your Being

This exercise takes you through the *koshas* on a journey of self-appreciation. Enjoy your physical form and the rolling waves of the breath. Truly appreciating physical and energetic forms connects us to the *Tantra* Path.

Step 1: Select a part of your body you appreciate. You may admire its strength, beauty, function, romantic association—it doesn't matter. The point is to find a part of your body you feel good about. It can be as large as a limb or torso or as small as the nail bed on your baby finger.

Step 2: Sit or recline in a comfortable position and attune to the depth, rhythm, and flow of your breath. You do not have to direct the breath in any way; simply watch it flow and let the breath breathe for your body.

Step 3: As you watch the breath, notice how good it feels to have this vital force flowing through you. No matter how much you relax and let go, the breath continues to roll like ocean waves … in again … out again … vitalizing … surrendering … nourishing … releasing …

Step 4: Once you have a sense of that relaxed pleasure in breathing, set your awareness to the part of your body you selected in step 1. Imagine breathing into and out of that part like a dolphin breathes through a blowhole. The breath still distributes through your body; however, the focus is on the exchange directly at your feel-good body part. You may imagine this in a variety of ways, such as in a cartoon, compared to scientific concepts, or as a movement pattern. If you are having trouble, just ask yourself, "If this could work for me, how might that happen?" and trust what follows.

Step 5: Continue witnessing the process for three to twelve minutes. Wrap up the practice by imagining that feel-good sense of the breath amplifying and circulating through your entire body.

Step 6: Express what you perceived in your breath-energy body. You may play with interpretive dance, color, hum, or however else you wish to express that pleasurable body appreciation and subtle flow.

Return to this kind of practice throughout the day, taking pleasure in your breath and body.

You may have noticed from the previous exercise that your more subtle layers are less obvious than most of what you encounter in the material world. When we begin to experience beyond the range of the everyday, we open our potential for expressive freedom. It may be redundant to say that the delicate is not dense; however, this is a key point on the *Tantra* Path. In order to connect to transcendent energies, we must be less attached to what we find in the material realm. The following section lets you explore beyond your five senses to open your creative perceptions.

How Many Senses Do You Have?

How do we learn about the world around us? Through what we see, hear, touch, taste, and smell. In fact, we become so reliant on our five senses to teach us about the world that we often forget how flawed they truly are. Remember, your eyes, ears, and other sense organs can only perceive within a limited range of experience. We can't hear dog whistles or see Wi-Fi signals, yet they exist. Thus, when we remember that there are many factors at play beyond what we can see, hear, touch, taste, and smell, we open ourselves to a more comprehensive view of the world. When we become less attached to what our senses tell us is real, we are free to explore different realms of reality. How creative is that?!

The *tantric* tradition reminds us that the material realm is an illusion (*maya*) and ultimate reality can only be contacted by a shift in perception, as discussed in chapter 7. The difference is that the *Raja* Path gives us a systematic process of cultivating a meditative mind, while the *Tantra* Path gives a thriving interaction with spirit via the material/energetic world.

The following exercise offers the opportunity to interface with the world beyond the experience of your five senses.

Exercise: Sensing Beyond the Senses

How many senses do we have beyond the classic five? I am not sure it's relevant. What are we sensing with, if not our five senses? The yogis would say "the source of our senses." We could play in these abstractions for the rest of the chapter, however, it may be more useful to delve into a direct experience of these ideas. Throughout the next exercise, remember that you are perceiving through a different filter than usual, so the information may

come to you in strange, faint, creative, or unexpected ways. If you are not accustomed to playing with energy, you may need to repeat this exercise several times before the epiphany happens. If you are interested in the *Tantra* Path, be patient, enjoy the journey, and *stick with it.*

Step 1: Sit or lie down in nature or near a living thing such as a tree, a flower, or rain. Close your eyes and attune to the natural movement of your breath. Don't direct the breath in any way; simply trust the breath's own intelligence and watch it flow.

Step 2: Go more deeply inward. As you witness the breath, appreciate the experience of it: it feels so good to breathe! You don't have to do anything—the motion of the breath just happens.

Step 3: Acknowledge that the energy of the breath is circulating through your entire body. Sense its presence in your torso, back, limbs, neck, face. You may especially feel it in places like your digits, lips, tailbone, low belly, or chest (major and minor *chakras*). You may sense the breath as imagery, sound, tingling, warmth, lightness, aroma, flavor. Do not judge your unique way of filtering these perceptions. Trust yourself and your imagination.

Step 4: When you have an internal sense of the breath-energy flow, imagine it broadening. Let your body, energy, senses, mind, etc., interpret this in their own way—the intention is to perceive or imagine the breath becoming more expansive. It fills you then shines out of you, extending through your pores and creating a beautiful field around your physical form. You may pause at this point and bask in the sense of being bigger than your body.

Step 5: When you have a visceral sense of the space beyond your physical form, imagine it broadening again, this time connecting to the natural object nearby. It can be fun to sense the other life form with your eyes closed, using internal experiences to glean information. It may also help to open your eyes and

connect via your physical sense before returning to the subtle connection. Be gentle and patient. Free yourself from expectations of how the information may come to you or what you may sense from the natural subject. Openness is important. Stay curious and connected as you trust your perceptions.

Step 6: Use this energetic connection as a perceptual bridge to gain a true sense of the natural item you are connecting with, all the while remaining energetically connected to the sense of your breath filling your physical form and expanding outward. You may pick up the simultaneously grounded and reaching actions of a tree, the bubbly freedom of a running stream, the fragility of flower petals, or the pent-up release of falling rain.

Step 7: When you are ready, offer appreciation to the living thing who shared your energetic space by smiling from your heart, saying a prayer, or sending gratitude. "Let go" of it. Begin to draw your presence back into your own energetic space, then into your body.

Step 8: Take your time awakening to the world around you. Use your five physical senses to experience yourself and your environment. You may notice that your sense organs are more sensitive now. Stay relaxed and witness the world with new eyes, so to speak.

Step 9: Express yourself as if you were the aspect of nature you were just connecting with. Write what the grounded, reaching tree might say. Paint the way the stream runs. Play piano with a flower petal's touch. Dance like a bursting cloud. Let your connection with the world guide your expression. You are a part of everything around you.

By connecting to your own body, then broadening that kinesthetic sense into the world around you, you gain a tender kind of access to the nuances of life. Continue appreciating the world

with this expanded sense of being. Being in nature is an essential aspect of staying balanced on the *Tantra* Path. Have you heard of a forest bath? It washes away the gritty stresses of the everyday, human-made world. Life feels different when we're in the thick of nature. We can perceive ourselves being nourished. This gentle, unified sense can greatly inform your creative process. In your creative life, you may apply this exercise to help you connect to movement in a visual piece or characterological aspects in your novel, film, or poem. We often perceive more than we think we do, even within the realm of the five senses, and attention to these details can be the thing that enhances our creative endeavors.

Sensing Intuition

As with the previous exercise, yoga offers a path to subtle-sense perceptions. When we are sensitive to our environments, we perceive more than the limited amount of information our five senses take in. Even within the range of what our senses record there are countless bits of information. It is possible that we are not even aware of all the content we are gathering, as the brain filters sensory "noise" from what is important and should be attended. The interesting thing is, all of the information the senses perceive is recorded on some level—it is just that most of it is not conscious!

Exercise: Become Conscious of What You Are Sensing

This practice helps you become more aware of the information your senses are picking up. This increases your sensitivity to yourself and the world around you while giving you greater access to creative nuance as you perceive the world more completely.

Step 1: Perform a typical task that does not require much attention, such as going for a walk, brushing your teeth, or washing dishes. As you do so, notice what you see, hear, taste, feel, and smell.

Step 2: Intend to become more aware. What else do you see, hear, taste, feel, and smell? If you are walking, you may notice the calls and colors of the birds around you, the feeling of the wind across your skin, and the smell of trees, ditches, lilacs, or car exhaust, in addition to how some of those smells linger in your mouth. You will notice the sensations as your muscles move and the feeling of your clothes on your skin, as well as the ground beneath you. You may hear barking dogs and cars going by (notice their colors, too, and how many people are in each car, and how fast they are driving), in addition to the continual sound of your own footfalls.

Step 3: Intensify that awareness again—there is still more to perceive! See how much you can notice at once.

Can you imagine what it would be like to be conscious of everything you saw, heard, smelled, tasted, touched in every moment? Potentially maddening, isn't it? There are *many* tidbits of information that we just do not need to give our focus to. What if you were aware of the feel of your clothing all day? It would be very distracting. The thing is, the nerves are still picking up and recording information about these unimportant perceptions continually. One of the implications of this is that we know far more about ourselves and our environments than we think we do. Accessing the greater awareness is an outcome of yoga practice. The following exercise offers you a practical experience of how to use that information hidden beyond your awareness.

Exercise: Tapping into Nonconscious Sensory Recordings

This is a simple practice to get you started. Note that you can elaborate this practice to tap into false core beliefs that may be holding you back or into unprocessed memories that may inspire your creative work. You will be guided to ask a question. Remember to stay relaxed and allow an answer to arise, rather than forcing an awareness. Your mind may jump in with doubts or attachments but your focus rests beyond that mental busyness in your nonconscious creative realms. This is an opportunity to use your creativity, as the response to your questions may come in the form of images, feelings, or some other cryptic answer. Trust what arises.

A Note of Caution: You know how in the olden days explorers hadn't gotten together to share what they knew about maps of the world? Instead, maps would note unexplored areas with the phrase "Here There Be Dragons." Our nonconscious realm is like that. We shove many dragons to the backs of our minds. Be gentle with yourself if you go exploring the depths, and I suggest you not go alone. Even a few counseling sessions can help keep you safe if any of those beasties happen to breathe fire. Sometimes there is deeper pain tucked away than we originally expect and, although it won't come out unless you are ready to process it, processing it can be tough.

Step 1: Name something you are stuck on—a question you haven't been able to answer or an item you have lost.

Step 2: Repeat steps 2, 3, and 4 from the Sensing Beyond the Senses exercise earlier in this chapter.

a. Once you have a sense of your vital force filling your body, imagine drawing it more deeply inward to the inception point of your ideas. It is okay if you don't really know where that is right now; just imagine going there and it will be so.

b. Once you have a sense of your vital force filling your body, imagine expanding it outward, through your skin into the cosmic realm or fourth dimension (space-time).

Step 3: As you settle into this space of creative potential, invite the solution to join you. This could be the next step regarding what you are stuck on, the answer to your lingering question, or a hint about what happened to your lost item. Ask the question once, clear and simple, then relax and note what arises.

Step 4: Call your energy back into your body, noticing the breath and physical sensations there, then follow your five senses into the material world your body occupies. Use whatever answer arises as the impetus for expressive work. You may whistle, draw, take immediate action in your life, or perform whatever other expressive method helps you elaborate and explore the answer that came.

Listen to Your Inner Voice

As the previous exercises may show, there is a part of you that is already connected to the vastness of creative possibility. Many of us are in the habit of getting in our own way: we don't trust the movement of the brush, the words in our orations, our next joke in the improv class. What would happen if you let these impulses out? The risk, I suppose, is failure, chaos, making a mistake; but, as already discussed, the potential rewards of trusting ourselves are enormous. A part of you already knows what it needs and where your brilliance is. Trust that sense. When it feels too hard to trust yourself, take a note from the *Karma* Path and do not be attached to the end result. It is a pleasure to let ourselves *be* ourselves and express that authentic being in as many ways as possible. Truly listening to and expressing from the inner voice is the deepest kind of connection the *Tantra* Path can give.

Exercise: Yoga Posture Practice: Connect with Your Natural Inner Aspects

The following yoga posture practice tunes you in to inherent aspects of yourself and gives you the chance to explore what it might be to live as other life-forms. Adapt the postures in whatever way you wish for your own comfort and safety. The important part is sensing new ways of being in the world, not how the pose looks from the outside. In this exercise, your body is a vehicle of exploration and insight.

Step 1: Select a quiet time of day and go to a park or along a nature trail. Walk briskly for at least three minutes to get yourself warmed up and ready for yoga postures.

Step 2: Stand in front of a tree that you find appealing. Imagine yourself growing roots from your low belly, through the perineum, down the insides of your legs and through the soles of your feet. Sense the warm earth, harder dirt, and bedrock. Notice as your roots spread how they interact with the roots of the tree in front of you and other plants in the area. Note the tree's strong trunk and feel that thick presence in your own stable torso as you pick one foot off the ground, turn the knee out to the side, and set the foot above or below the knee of the opposite leg. Staying grounded, follow that upward sense of energy through the strong torso and spine, lifting the crown of the head. You may grow your arms like branches to the sky, letting yourself form the kind of tree that you are (evergreen, maple, birch …). Continue connecting with the tree in front of you and sensing what it is like to be part of a forest. When ready, trade sides. You may repeat this a few times.

Step 3: Find a running stream or fountain. Take some time to listen to the melody of the running water and note its fluid freedom. When ready, bend forward from the hips and pour your torso over the front of your thighs. Bend your knees as much as you need to in order to feel a sense of letting go through the upper body and fold forward. Arms and head can hang loosely. Feel as though your upper body were running water, mobile and free, as it cascades forward and down like water running over the cliff face of your legs.

Step 4: Note the birds. See how their chests are full and round and the way their wings spread wide as they soar. Some birds walk by moving their heads forward first, then walking their feet forward in line with the head. Spread your feet wide. You may bend your knees out over your toes, and combine the following birdlike actions:

a. Puff your chest up, creating a bend in your thoracic spine. Feel your shoulders roll back as you press your heart forward/up.

b. Spread your wings (arms) wide to the sides, feeling light and open.

c. Slide your chin forward. You may purse your lips and open and close your "beak."

d. You can stick out your tail feathers, creating an even arch through your entire spine. Perceive yourself as a creature of the sky, able to take off and see things from higher perspectives at any time.

Step 5: Gather some stones/twigs and, if there is one nearby, go sit cross-legged on a boulder (or dangle your legs off the side if you can't cross them). Stack the stones/twigs one on top of the other, creating a spiraling action. Notice that each item is just a little bit twisted from the one below it, but the top twig/stone is far more revolved than its foundation. Imagine this stack of natural objects represents your spine and spiral yourself into a seated twisting pose. Remain erect as you rotate through abdomen, ribs, shoulders, and neck to look over your back shoulder, perceiving the revolving motion of your spinal column and the energy within. Repeat on the other side. You may practice this posture a few times each side.

Step 6: Observe the arc of a blade of grass growing from the ground in a gentle bend. Plant your feet together or shoulder-width apart, reach your arms overhead, palms together or apart, and bend yourself sideward to the left, then right. Perceive your body as a small living thing, easily influenced by the weather around it yet diligent in its growth as it reaches for the sun. You may go through this action a few times, aligning yourself with the tender strength of plant life.

Step 7: Based on this *asana* practice of connecting with nature, create an artistic piece. You may write from the point of view of your natural objects, or draw what they see from their vantage point, or move with their motivation and quality of action.

Anytime you feel stuck in your creative process, return to your senses and the natural world around you, drawing inspiration from the connection between the inner and outer world.

Trust Yourself

The *Tantra* Path shows that when we are truly connected—whether to our own spirit or nature or in a collaborative project—connection provides a genuine sense of spiritual resonance. A key point of this chapter is that you are connected to forces beyond your wee body and human power. You are made of stardust. (It's true; look it up.) You have access to more realms of the human condition and your own unexplored territory than could fill a library of books or films, a gallery of paintings or sculptures, or myriad festivals of song and dance. You are already a part of everything you need to create authentic, truthful, brilliant expressions. Follow your breath, your connection to life, and your intuitive sense, and enjoy the process of expressing that which is greater than your everyday experience. Feel it!

Now you have the chance to play with the idea that creation is enlightenment. Yoga offers five paths to access the enlightened, creative Self. *Karma* is that path of purpose in creation. We can follow the system that *Raja* Yoga gives us and apply the eight limbs to our creative process. The *Bhakti* Path, the path of the heart, helps us move through old pain so that we are free to be tender, joyful, and imaginative. The path of *Jnana* is an intellectual one: observing, researching, and theorizing. The *Tantra* Path approaches creativity through the body-energy-mind. Continue to play with all five paths while honoring the ones that you are predisposed to.

The next section of this book attunes to your neurological makeup and how the brain can either help or hinder our creative lives.

Part 3
Creative Living with Yoga & Expressive Arts

WE CONCLUDE *Yoga for the Creative Soul* with a journey through the brain. So far you have explored what stands between you and your true, creative Self and then explored various paths to connect with your creative essence. Now you are going to explore your anatomical brain and the ways its structure and function can inhibit or support your creative process.

As with the previous two parts of this book, part 3 offers you diverse, practical expressive arts and yoga therapy exercises. The focus of this section is your neuroanatomy and how you can use brain science to be more creative. Read on, and enjoy this section as it supports you in removing the obstacles that stand between you and a connection to your creative zest for life. You can explore the beliefs, experiences, and proclivities that limit your free expression and apply creative practices to learn more about why these barriers interfere with your unique personal journey. You will notice that some obstacles possess more power than others. It is okay for you to experiment with different barriers to different degrees on different days. Sometimes you may wish to examine deep, personal challenges and other times take a gentle path to getting more insight about what you already have a handle on. Revisit part 1 anytime you lose touch with your creative process, as a means of removing what may be standing in your way. Be playful and accepting—there is no right or wrong way to create. This is your journey. Enjoy it!

Your reptilian, mammalian, and human brains work together with your creative soul to offer you a life of brilliant inspiration. Part 3 guides you in creating joy in everyday life through your unique brand of self-expression. Experiment with bringing color, movement, and melody into daily routines, rooms of the home, work life, and personal relationships. You may be especially interested in the segment on global creativity: your ability to effect change on a larger scale via your creative efforts. Creative living improves your brain health and psychological functioning and is instrumental in disease prevention/healing. Peel back the following pages and find out how.

Chapter 11
The Reptilian Brain & Your Base Instincts

THINK ABOUT YOUR BRAIN. (Is that your brain's form of self-reflection?) Most multicellular organisms have brains; reptiles, mammals, birds, and amphibians have brains. Humans possess the most evolved of animal brains, and we can use our brains differently than any other animal that we are aware of.

Some scientists have an interesting model of vertebrate neuroevolution. Stay with me—this is neat-o. The idea is that the human brain can be viewed as three distinct brains, each with its own abilities and associated needs and behaviors. The three brains are reptilian, or hindbrain; paleomammalian, or limbic brain; and neomammalian, the neocortex. This three-part brain offers us a model through which we can also view our creative needs and effectiveness. This chapter focuses on the hindbrain and how caring for and heeding impulses from this reptilian aspect of your neurology can enhance your creative life.

The Reptilian Brain Needs...

The reptilian brain, sometimes called the hindbrain, is the most basic aspect of our neurology. You can find it at the top of your spine in the back (hence the term "hindbrain"). It includes the brain stem and cerebellum and governs your body's automatic processes, like beating your heart and keeping you breathing. Basically, it keeps us alive. The impetus to meet our basic survival needs comes from this brain.

What happens when our basic biological needs are not met? Life starts to feel very difficult when we are too hungry or tired. If you have ever watched a starving animal, you know it will fight with its life for food. Reptiles will protect their mates from competitors with fierce aggression. In our own way, the same is true for us. How well do you handle stress if you haven't had enough sleep? How motivated are you to dance, cook a proper meal, or spin a tale if you aren't fed or rested?

When our basic needs are not met, we are far more likely to be lazy (*tamasic*), inactive, and deferential to the outside world rather than to our true voice. We turn away from the inner creative impulses and rely on addictive feel-goods like alcohol, caffeine, TV, or the Internet. These issues are compounded over time, as our addictive tendencies are typically driven by the reptilian brain, which likes routine, consistency, and hedonism. After all, it can't think; what does it know about better options and a sense of meaning and fulfillment?

The reptilian brain is needs-focused. It has no forethought. Common scientific wisdom indicates that not only can it not think, it is actually in a dream state *at all times*. (Fortunately, our own limbic brain and neocortex suppress most of this constant dreaming.) The hindbrain perceives the world only through its own limited, surreal frame of reference. The following exercise gives you the chance to examine how well you are able to balance your relationship with lifestyle and your reptilian brain, in the form of a fun quiz.

 Exercise: Quiz: Is Your Reptilian Brain the Boss of You?

Answer the following questions as truthfully as possible by circling either *T* for true or *F* for false (or write your answers on a separate piece of paper). If you are not sure how to answer because you "sometimes" act that way, consider what you do 80 to 95 percent of the time and let that be your answer. Less than 80 percent of the time, go the other way. At the end of the quiz, add up all your "false" answers.

Hindbrain Habit

I get more than seven hours sleep per night .... T / F

I limit my unhealthy habits .... T / F

I stay relaxed when someone is eyeing my mate .... T / F

I am a generous person .... T / F

I have broken many unhealthy habits and not
    returned to them .... T / F

I generally trust others .... T / F

I eat till I am a little bit full, then stop............................... T / F

I am *not* easily distracted by sensory information .... T / F

I am comfortable with the unknown .... T / F

I acknowledge when I need a little rest............................... T / F

I notice when I am beginning to feel hungry...................... T / F

I readily share my belongings, food, and time.................... T / F

I am rarely jealous .... T / F

When people are near my home, such as walking
    past on the sidewalk, I can let it be without
    watching them through the window .... T / F

I handle conflict without being offensive or defensive .... T / F

I go with the flow... T / F

I don't worry about the future.. T / F

I can deviate from my routine without
    becoming stressed .... T / F

I prefer a moderate path to all-or-nothing approaches ...... T / F

I think through my options before making decisions .... **T / F**

I am flexible with my habits, routines, and behaviors .... **T / F**

I am able to suppress my desire for things I would
   really like to indulge in .... **T / F**

I don't yell, even when I am furious with the
   person in front of me .... **T / F**

In competitions, I am content even if my team loses.......... **T / F**

I don't mind when others are in control of the situation.... **T / F**

If you answered "false" to more than thirteen of the statements in this quiz, your reptilian brain might be running the show. You may benefit from acknowledging your basic requirements and their source more thoughtfully. Please do your best to care for your physical needs as they arise. When you are facing a desire or urge, rather than a true biological need, you may imagine soothing your inner reptile. The following exercise offers one way to do that.

Exercise: Relaxation to Calm Your Base Instincts

When we are stressed out, our most basic urges take over and we lose touch with the creative Self. Spending just a bit of time on relaxation can help soothe the reptilian brain and reset your inspiration.

Step 1: Lie down on your mat on your abdomen in Crocodile Pose (*Makarasana*): big toes together, heels rolled to the outsides, and forehead or cheek placed on the back of your hands/folded arms. Now you are resting comfortably on your stomach. Perceive the good feeling of your breath against the floor. Notice how each time you exhale, the ground conspires with you to press the lungs empty, allowing a sense of surrender.

Step 2: Imagine yourself as you are right now, as if looking from the outside. See your resting form with genuine compassion and care. As you continue to regard yourself, begin to imagine your devolution. The image of yourself shifts from a human to a creature, then this creature forms the shape of a lizard. Imagine your legs as the lizard's tail, your spine and head where it would be. Continue breathing deeply and gazing upon this animal with compassion.

Step 3: Imagine the lizard's impulses: how much it wants to eat, warm itself, rest, and be safe. Understand that the lizard feels safest when held in its own familiar routines. Sometimes there are options *outside* the realm of what it truly needs that it gets used to having, and even though these things do not support its safety or survival (in fact, some may be leading the lizard to an early death), the lizard continues to partake. Hold compassion for the automatic processes of the lizard. Remember that it has no ability to control its impulses, no option to think ahead and understand why it might choose to.

Step 4: After you have relaxed with the image of the lizard for a time, offering it compassionate, objective understanding, imagine the lizard morphing back into a human. As you witness the change within yourself, imagine what is happening within the cranium. Perceive that just as the body is becoming more human, so the brain is developing, wrapping layers of connections around that basic reptilian brain, adding in a conscience, goals, and sense of Self as well as future Self.

Step 5: Let the human connect with its inner lizard and take what meaning it can from the lizard's impulses and desires. As a more thoughtful creature, how can the base desires be transformed into something uplifting, healthy, and inspiring for yourself/others? For example, if your urge for cake brought you to this exercise and you perceived your lizard tasting an immediate sense of sweetness—unknowing that the cake will cause gain weight, clog arteries, create inflammation, burn out the pancreas, etc.—how can the human-you offer your lizard a more genuine and lasting sense of sweetness in life? The same question can be asked of the escape via drugs, the pick-me-up of caffeine, the validation of sex, the thrill of pornography, the safe connections through social media, or the distraction of passive entertainment.

Step 6: Express the human alternative to the lizard's impulsive need. You may write a dialogue between the brains, display the transformation through interpretive dance, or even create the alternative itself, such as in the form of a healthy meal or prayer.

Use this exercise anytime you feel as if your selfish, most basic instincts are driving you and limiting your connection to the creative Self.

Feeeed Meeee!

Modern culture has some issues with food. In many cases it is an issue of information overload. There is a plethora of conflicting, scientifically validated studies about the best way to eat: grazing versus two large meals per day, vegan versus paleo, low-fat versus high-fat, and many other confusing contradictions. When we are not feeding ourselves properly, whether out of confusion, busyness, disorder, or whatever, the nervous system is too stressed to rest into a creative state. A yogic approach to nutrition, which is also scientifically validated, is learning about and meeting your own body's needs via mindfulness.

 Exercise: Insight & Mindful Awareness

Mindfulness is the common term for awareness, witnessing, or insight. The following exercise is a beginning mindfulness practice.

Step 1: Sit or stand comfortably. Commit to not judging yourself, wishing things were different, or trying to change what is. This practice is about becoming conscious of what is there, not making it any different.

Step 2: Notice the sensations in your body: the feeling of the air around you, clothes against your skin, ground holding you up, coupled with inner sensations such as muscular tightness and relaxation, physical comfort or discomfort, heart rate, and the movement of your breath.

Step 3: Become more aware of your breath. How is it moving (smoothly, choppily, erratically, deeply, shallowly, etc.)? Where is it in your body? What else is notable?

Step 4: Deepen your emotional awareness. How are you feeling? Which emotions are present? Some may be comfortable or uncomfortable—they might even be in opposition to one another. It's okay—just notice.

Step 5: Witness the thoughts moving through your mind. Acknowledge what you are thinking without trying to direct your thoughts; just watch them pass and be aware of their content. Sometimes when we watch our thoughts they get faster at first. This is normal—just keep watching. After a few minutes, go on about your day. You can become mindful again whenever you wish and during any task.

Exercise: Awareness at Mealtime

You can bring mindfulness to any moment in life. When we are conscious of our internal realm, it is easier to create from a place of inner truth. We also have greater access to our inner well of inspiration. When you apply mindfulness practice to eating, you are less likely to overeat or choose foods that have a negative impact on your health. You are more likely to enjoy complete, healthy digestion, including comfortable, timely elimination and better absorption of nutrients from your food. Mindfulness will support you in knowing when you are hungry, so you can readily honor the needs of your body, and when you are full, so you avoid consuming more than is healthy for you. Before your next meal, review and apply this Mindful Eating exercise.

Step 1: Set your meal in front of you. (Note: For a better sense of precision and nuance with your food, you may complete this exercise with a single food item, such as a piece of fruit or vegetable or anything you may consume on a habitual basis.) Observe the food up close. Notice the visible colors and textures, the balance and form of your plate, the way you might admire a painting in a gallery. Similar to the gallery experience, also take a few steps back and observe your plate from a distance the way you would regard a fine work of art.

Step 2: Sit down in front of your plate and regard it again. "We eat with our eyes first." Feel your body and breath relax as you focus on the aromas wafting from your meal. Spend some time with these scents, seeing if you can discern the separate ingredients and also notice the fragrance as a complete unit. What does the smell of your food inform you about its flavor? Can you tell if your body is readying itself for a meal? If so, how?

Step 3: If possible, pick your food up with your fingers; otherwise, lift it upon your fork and gaze at it for a breath or two. What happens within you as you anticipate taking this bite? This is a distinct difference between the refined eating habits of a human and that of a reptilian beast. Savor the moment between your plate and your palate.

Step 4: Before putting the food in your mouth (I know it seems like this is taking forever—you'll thank me later), allow it to interact with your lips. Our lips are one of the most sensitive parts of the body. What do they tell you about the texture of this food? Lick any residual flavors from your lips and notice the response of your taste buds, mind, stomach, salivary glands, and other body parts.

Step 5: Don't bite it yet, but place the food in your mouth. Now what do you notice about its texture, flavor, and aroma? What is it like to roll it around in your mouth? Do different parts of your mouth perceive it differently?

Step 6: The moment you've been waiting for: bite into your meal! What do you experience as your teeth sink through the food? Is the texture what you expected? Are there more nuances of flavor? As you continue to chew, let the food sit on different parts of your tongue. Does location shift the nature of the flavor or your ability to enjoy the food? How about chewing on the left or right side? Did any emotions accompany the act of chewing?

Step 7: Once you have fully masticated so that the solid food has been liquefied into a bolus, swallow. Observe the process of moving food from the mouth, through the esophagus. Can you tell how your stomach receives this morsel?

Step 8: Continue with this process as much as possible. Anytime you notice your mind wandering from the food or an impulse to speed up your eating, bring yourself back to any of the previous steps. Remain aware and measured in pace as you ingest your meal, one conscious bite at a time.

Step 9: Even if there is still some food left on your plate, stop eating when you feel satiated. The *Kundalini Upanishad* recommends having the stomach half full of food, quarter full of nutritious liquid like lassi, and quarter full of air to allow room for digestion. In other words, eat until you are content, not stuffed. When you are free from your reptilian mind and fear of lack, you can remember that when you get hungry again, you will eat again;

it's okay if you are not "stuffed." Take a few breaths and notice how you feel following the meal. Is it easy to breathe deeply? Where does your breath want to go in your body? What is the speed and quality of your thoughts? How did this meal affect your sense of relaxation, well-being, and enthusiasm?

Step 10: Check in with yourself an hour after the meal and again after two hours, as well as before bed, upon rising, and each time you use the toilet. Acknowledge the effects of your eating behavior and food choices.

Practice eating this way for a week or three and notice shifts in your metabolism, state of mind, addictive tendencies, elimination, energy level, body shape, and creative inspiration. When we feed ourselves properly, whether through mindfulness habits or other nutrition strategies, we feel safer in the world. This sense of safety lets the reptile within us rest so that we can focus on higher aspects of our lives such as self-expression and spiritual growth. Please do not underestimate the importance of balanced eating in your creative life.

Rest Is Best

Balanced sleeping habits are another undervalued aspect of creative living. This is especially true because of the typical lifestyle habits of a creative person, such as following inspiration into the wee hours of the morning and living outside of structured daily routines. Whether or not you fall prey to those habits, if you are living in modern society there are likely issues with your sleep.

Electric lights have made it easy for us to override our healthy circadian rhythms. Ambient light in our bedrooms, even after we have cut all the lights, alters our melatonin levels and interferes with deep sleep. Blue screens, sugar, caffeine, cigarettes, stress, and poor coping strategies and bedtime routines all play together in making our overnight time less effective and restful than we need. As we cultivate a habit of overriding our feelings of fatigue, we also cultivate lethargy, dis-ease, and disconnection.

Consider the possibility that going to bed when it is dark and getting up when it is light can have a huge impact on your creative resources and flow of ideas. How many strokes of genius have arisen in the twilight between sleeping and waking, the restfulness of a warm bath, or the bizarre and brilliant dreamscape? When you feel depleted and like you are losing your creative essence, go lie down. Turn off your devices; shut off the noise and go rest with yourself. If your stresses creep in with you, apply the basic mindfulness practice or lizard transformation practice from earlier in this chapter. Alternatively, you may enjoy the following practice.

Exercise: Rest/Relax in Safety

This practice is useful if you need rest or are stressed. Use the power of sense memory to connect to the calm purity of nature.

Step 1: Lie down somewhere you will not be disturbed for an extended period of time. If there is somewhere you have to be later, set an alarm then free your mind from all sense of responsibility for the time being. Suggest that your body and breath relax and trust them to continue to do so.

Step 2: Imagine yourself in nature. This can be a place wholly of your own creation, somewhere you once encountered, or a favorite place you like to visit. Experience this place with all of your being. How does the air smell? Can you hear water, rustling trees, or birds nearby? What is the time of day, the temperature, the landscape? As you continue to relax in this quiet, natural space, fill in as many details as possible.

Step 3: You may rest here for as long as you wish, or follow the comfort and safety of this space into sleep.

Who's In Charge Here?

As you get to know your hindbrain and base instincts better, you are less likely to fall prey to outside influences. This can mean great gains in your creative, financial, and romantic lives. The reptilian brain orients itself around safety and survival. Another way of saying this is that it operates from a space of selfishness and fear. When we are afraid, we tend to stop considering others. This includes those who are closest to us but is especially noticeable in society at large. Marketing is fear-based, so we buy products instead of donating that excess to worthy charities. We may spend money we don't have to "keep up with the Joneses," which creates the insecurity of debt which in turn has us working jobs we don't like rather than spending that time on creative or more fulfilling career pursuits. The reptilian brain, and those who know how to manipulate it, pose grand obstacles to our creative Selves.

The antidote for this is to continue to cultivate safety and trust our own frame of reference. Build community with others who value self-expression and creativity and spend at least a little time and money on causes that call to your heart. When we operate from the reptilian brain, we become incapable of bonding together in community, which in turn limits the potential impact that a collective of artists can have on others.

It is worth noting that when we are in times of challenging transition, crisis, or other extreme circumstances, the reptilian brain and its survival focus is a great tool. The rougher things become in everyday life, the more we can hold on to a sense of Self through maintaining routines and caring for ourselves in the most fundamental ways. Beyond those times when we are in survival mode, however, deference to the reptilian brain makes us less of who we really are and limits our potential to know ourselves, grow, and inspire.

We get out of the hindbrain by caring for ourselves, trusting our ability to survive, and in turn cultivating hope, faith, nourishment, and connection to Self—beyond selfishness—and others. The reptilian brain is responsible for survival. Once you know you are confident in survival, you can move on to higher realms and express your creative Self more fully.

Chapter 12
Play Is a Need

NOW THAT WE HAVE carried ourselves beyond the survival mode of the reptilian brain, we can move on to a discussion of the paleomammalian (PM), or midbrain. The midbrain is our emotional center and the location of many automatic reactions. It does not involve itself in higher reasoning, which I will visit in the next chapter. In this chapter, think of yourself more as a puppy, with immediate needs and reactions, than an enlightened creator.

The PM brain is composed of the hippocampus, hypothalamus, and amygdala. The hippocampus is associated with memory, especially long-term, and some spatial abilities. The hypothalamus is very busy maintaining homeostatic balance throughout the body and coordinates with the hormonal and nervous systems. The amygdala is associated with emotional expression and learning about extreme emotions in order to respond more appropriately next time. Because of its role in ensuring survival, it is highly associated with fear and aggression.

Researchers are beginning to explore the role of the hippocampus, hypothalamus, and amygdala of the paleomammalian brain in creativity. Findings indicate that our emotional centers may inspire creative works and the PM brain supports creative thinking when we take proper care of ourselves, but, apart from some interesting findings about the amygdala (emotional expression), the PM brain does not play a direct role in creativity. Interestingly, in conditions where we feel threatened, the amygdala signals back into the hindbrain to tell the lizard that all is not well. On the other hand, when we feel safe, seen, and cared for, the amygdala is more likely to signal forward into the forebrain (higher reason) and help promote creative thinking.

In order to keep the PM brain balanced, we need our physiological and emotional needs cared for. Similar to the hindbrain, the midbrain also needs to feel safe; however, this higher PM brain includes emotional safety along with the basic biological needs the reptilian brain is concerned with. Nourishing the PM brain with self-care activities and community support sustains our overall enlightenment by ensuring that our more basic needs are met and increasing its connectivity with the forebrain and centers associated with higher thought. The following exercise helps you clarify specific ways you can tend to your own PM brain.

Exercise: Accessing the Creative Potential in Stored Emotions

There is great potential stored in the part of your brain that harbors emotions. Oftentimes, we do not process our painful experiences all the way to resolution. What this means is that the brain and nervous system still carry those impressions of pain. They still affect us. The good news is, we can continue processing those old feelings and experiences through creative expression. Follow the next exercise to experiment with connecting to that old pain. Remember to check in with your therapist before and after, especially if you have past trauma. Go gently with yourself and, even though this is about letting old wounds express, it is also meant to be fun. Stay mindful and witness the process objectively.

Step 1: Think of something that scared you in the past that you now avoid. Your amygdala helped teach you to do that. Even now while you are thinking about it, your amygdala is probably connecting with your reptilian brain. This is happening from sheer habit and you can train it to connect to the forebrain instead. Keep yourself safe and work with a memory that you have already processed a bit, not something that will trigger a traumatic incident. If you choose something from your traumatic history, make sure you have an appointment lined up with your therapist and a crisis line number nearby in case you need to process.

Step 2: Using the personal example from step 1, identify the *beneficial* lessons that arose from that frightening situation. What did you learn about yourself? Did anything lovely arise, either directly or indirectly, as a result of it?

Step 3: The amygdala helped you process the intense emotions that surrounded that frightening thing, in addition to training you to avoid it in the future. Let's tap into those old emotions and channel them into your creative resources. Without applying any language and with the grounding help of your breath, grab a crayon, or, if you can make a big mess, a paintbrush in each hand and move your body in a way that "describes" the intense feelings. Maybe your arms flail. Perhaps you punch or stab the canvas. You can spin or jump or slash while you express. You may make some sounds. Do your best to stay connected to your breath and present in the moment. You are completely safe and *choosing* to use this old fear as an impetus for creativity. Remember that this is only a page or canvas and your physical expression will not cause harm to anyone else. This is a private moment between you, your brain, and your emotions.

Step 4: When you have spent your expression, give yourself a gentle, loving reward of some kind (the amygdala loves these). Soak in a hot bath, massage your skull, or do one of the relaxations from this book. Affirm that you are physically secure now and it is safe to feel and express your emotions.

You may return to this exercise in times when your creative well has run dry. Our old pains offer a wealth of expressive potential. The initial, raw material might not be the beautiful product you are looking for but it is so real that new expressive styles and inspirations arise. It has the added benefit of altering your neural patterns and connecting you more deeply with your enlightened Self while decoupling old connections to that selfish lizard hindbrain.

An overactive amygdala is associated with anxiety, which in turn limits our creative potential. Anxiety narrows our attention and keeps us looking at life through the eyes of fear. The only thing anxiety helps us create is more fear and visions of all the things that could go wrong. I offer a wealth of exercises and insights about transforming anxiety into confidence in *Yoga Therapy for Stress and Anxiety*. By transcending your anxious habits, you free yourself to explore more diverse and authentic modes of self-expression.

 Exercise: Find Your Tribe

We feel safer and more engaged in expressing ourselves when connected with like-minded others. This community mindedness is a fundamental mammalian need. The PM brain perceives social rejection as a physical threat. Let this exercise help you find ways to seek out and connect with your people.

Step 1: You've already been doing this step throughout the book: step 1 is "Get to know your true Self." Learn about what you believe, what is important to you, what you enjoy, how you interact with the world, who you wish to be.

Step 2: You've been doing this one, too: understand what is going on beneath the programs that run in your mind and, as you deprogram, express yourself more freely and fully. As we are truthful in our self-expression, those who are like us harmonize with that and join in.

Step 3: Have you been doing this one yet? Get out there! Your tribe is not going to come to you if you hide behind closed doors. No one is saying "Let's get over to 1368 Burdock Ave. Jo is crooning melodies that would bring tears to our eyes. We'll feel so seen!" No. Your tribe, for the most part, is hiding behind their own closed doors. I believe that the more we create or join clubs, attend meet-ups/workshops/retreats, and support local spiritual, artistic, social, and political endeavors, the more others will do the same. Through this action, we find one another.

Step 4 (Optional): If you are more of an introverted type, as both yogis and creatives often are, you may wish to be more discerning about how you get out there. Some folks do very well with trial-and-error (going to anything and everything then leaving if it isn't their scene). If for whatever reason you find it harder to get out of the house, try this:

a. Peruse local television stations, libraries, crafting stores, music shops, coffee houses, newspapers, dance or yoga studios, e-zines, tourist sites, Facebook events, high school and college websites, and www.meetup.com to explore options that pique your interest. Be sure to jot down all your ideas on a comprehensive list.

b. Review your list and circle three to five events you find most enticing, inspiring, or appealing.

c. Commit to attending an average of one per week. If that feels like too much, try one per month, or each time loneliness feels overwhelming.

d. Invite a friend to go with you if it helps you get out there.

Finding your tribe takes effort and it is totally worth it. The more we express our authentic selves, the less we fit a typical societal mold. Nobody likes or needs to feel lonely. There is actually a neurological cost to isolation, not to mention the emotional ones. Many people will resonate with you, but it does take some effort to find them. The more we venture out of our houses to things that truly call us, the more we will discover and connect with one another. I hope you come out and play soon!

Play

I once ran a retreat about healing trauma and related the three brains to yoga therapy principles that help us overcome a painful past. In that workshop, the group brainstormed fundamental mammalian needs: survival basics, community, touch, love, order, leadership … It wasn't long before they started repeating themselves, but they missed one key need. "There's something you're forgetting … think of your dog."

"Food!" "Discipline!" "Exercise!" They couldn't come up with it. After ten minutes, I left the room and told them to relax and think about it. "Could you just tell us?" they asked.

I said, "The reason I'm not telling you is I need you to understand how far off your radar this is."

Eventually, someone thought of *play*. We went outside and had recess for grown-ups. Some played Frisbee; others kicked a soccer ball around. A small group played hide-and-go-seek. I highly recommend it.

Many adults have forgotten how to play, or they think that we aren't supposed to. As you connect to your creative essence and child self, you will become clearer and clearer on the importance of play. Some of the most enlightened people on our planet are incredibly playful. Have you heard the Dalai Lama laugh? He does it all the time! As we connect more deeply to our spiritual selves, it's easier to take most of life in stride. As we open to the creative Self, we perceive more opportunities to enjoy life. The more open our minds and hearts, the more we can see the humor and lightheartedness in all things.

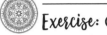

Exercise: Grown-Up Playtime

This exercise reminds you of some ways to play as an adult. After years of being programmed to work hard, achieve, and fit in, it can take some time to get back in touch with our playful selves. Cultivating a playful attitude keeps us creative. This is especially true if you come from a rigid or violent home, or had to grow up too soon. Even if it makes you feel uncomfortable at first, seek out some fun and playfulness.

Step 1: Remember what you did for fun when you were three or four years old? How about eight or ten? Did you ever play creative games? Even sculpting dough, coloring books, and paint-by-numbers give hints about your early creative aptitudes and interests.

Step 2: Remember the last time you let loose and had fun. I don't necessarily mean being raucous or a troublemaker—just clean, happy times. If you can't remember, you aren't alone. Many adults have had the fun "lifed" right out of them. Even if it was thirty years ago, remember.

Step 3: Remember that life is meant to be fun and there are playful opportunities all around you right now. Yes, now. Look.

Step 4: List activities that make you feel giddy, free, safe, and invigorated. Can you be silly? Prove it.

Step 5 (optional): If you need help busting out of your stoic self, spend the next hour speaking complete gibberish. Don't do this at work, but at home it is a safe activity. It is much more amusing to do it with others, though. Call up a silly or creative friend and tell them you want to practice a new language and they can join in. You may be amazed to find that after a few minutes of gibberish, you begin to understand one another.

Your amygdala is so happy that you are remembering the intense emotion of "fun." Even if you have trouble playing as an adult, there are many opportunities out there. There's play in *asana* and most other forms of movement. There's play in just putting on music and doing what your body wants to do. The swing set is always good for adults, even if all you do is sit on a swing and rock gently. If your wrists will tolerate cartwheels, keep cartwheeling. Or do somersaults in the pool. Speak in a funny voice or wear outrageous clothes. Look for the joke in everything; it's always there.

Spend as much time as possible with people who make you laugh. Find ways to make others laugh. Continue saying yes to fun and playful opportunities. As you do, enjoy the way it improves your health and point of view, as well as making life itself feel more like a creative act. Speaking of playing like grown-ups and creative acts, what about sex?

Shagging

Birds do it; bees do it; it's natural. Some yogis practice abstinence (*brahmacharya*) as an aspect of their spirituality. This is to direct sexual energy toward the sacred. Most people in today's society, however, are sexually active. Sex can be a spiritual practice that connects us to our creative essence more deeply. See for yourself via the following exercise.

Exercise: Spiritual Sex

This exercise is for any sexual person. You do not need a partner to perform this. Follow the steps and enjoy a sexual form of play.

Step 1: Select a partner. This can be a consensual partner, the divine, your own body, or an idea/concept such as possibility, infinity, or creativity.

Step 2: Spend quiet time meditating or communing with your partner. Practices such as intentional breath, eye gazing, or sounding are excellent connectors. Keep a delicate smile on your face and beaming through your eyes. Although you are sincere, do not be serious.

Step 3: Pay attention to the subtle realms as you activate more sexual, pleasurable feelings. Be aware of breath, thoughts, shared emotions, and a continual sense of connection.

Step 4: As pleasure heightens, continue feeding it back into your original intention. Remain relaxed and happy. Do not get caught in a personal agenda or thought of outcome. Be present to the subtleties of what is happening by keeping step 3 vital. If you feel the peak coming, take a break or repeat step 2. Be playful, silly, and joyful about this experience. Allow your whole personality to shine through as you connect with inner (and outer) divinity via pleasure.

Step 5 (optional): After delaying gratification a few times, head into climax with faith that you are approaching a divine moment. Through connection with your chosen partner, perceive a launch into transcendent space. As you prolong this expansion (the more times you repeat step 4, typically, the longer you will bask in step 5), be intentional about the divine qualities you are contacting. As the peaking waves begin to subside, be clear about what divine qualities or future possibilities you draw from this pure well of goodness. Trust that you are integrating them into yourself.

Step 6: Whether you stopped at step 4 or 5, spend some time relaxing and integrating the experience. Focus on the intentions and qualities you carried with you during this playful, pleasurable time. Imagine them weaving into your being. The next time you embark upon a creative endeavor, call these qualities forth.

Sex may be the original creative act. When approached properly, it can connect us to higher creation and our own creative potential. We waste energy when we indulge in disconnected or addictive sex. We cultivate purpose and inspiration when we approach it intentionally. Its power can support all of our endeavors. Sex, however, is not necessary if you are abstinent. The following platonic practice gives you similar access to connection, play, and creativity.

Exercise: Yoga Posture Practice: Playful Partner Poses

This exercise invites more laughter and connection into your life. Repeat it with as many different people as possible. Feel welcome to try some of your own favorite yoga poses with a partner, too.

Step 1: Invite a friend, loved one, or pet to practice some simple yoga postures with you (you get to be extra creative if you are working with a pet). Enjoy the experience of being creative and playful together. This isn't an exercise regime (although that is another fun way to play); rather, it is a chance to explore movement and touch in the context of a healthful practice. Go for a quick walk or do some gentle movements to warm up.

Step 2: Spine/Breath Connection—Set your yoga mats with the long edges together or find a clean floor or grassy lawn to play on. Begin by sitting back-to-back. Notice how you hold one another up. This is a nice connection! As you let your own breath deepen, also sense your partner's breath deepening. What happens if you try to coordinate your breathing patterns?

Step 3: Forward/Backward Bend—Extend your legs out in front of you, in line with the hips or in a wide V-shape. Without making a verbal agreement, sense which partner is going to lean back and which will lean forward. Observe how you negotiate the movement without using your words. Be gentle so each person is able to stop when they have leaned forward/backward far enough. How do you know it is time to come out of the pose and switch?

Step 4: Twist—If your legs are crossed, cross them the other way. If they are straight, widen the distance between the feet. If they are already wide, great. Link elbows with your partner and sit tall. Do your best to keep the backs of your shoulders connected to one another as you rotate to one side. Move slowly so no one gets pushed beyond healthy limits. Without speaking, decide together when it is time to twist to the other side. You may repeat this action a few times and even try it standing up. Stay playful. Are there ways to joke around without using words?

Step 5: Side Bending—Come to standing, if you aren't already, and once again settle back-to-back. Straighten your arms out to the sides and have the taller partner bring the arms overtop so that you can place each palm against your partner's. With hands, heels, and backs united, begin bending from side-to-side, keeping the arms to the sides. If you are feeling very playful, you may make airplane noises and experiment with bending in different directions, such as forward, backward, or diagonally, as well. How does laughter effect the flow of movements and the postures themselves?

Step 6: Balance—Stand side-by-side, hip-to-hip, facing the same direction as your partner, with an arm around each other's waists. Outside arm can go anywhere. Ground through the foot of the inside (partner side) leg. Each partner lifts the outside knee. Stabilize against each other's standing leg/torso as you bring your outside knees to hip height in front of you. Help each other stay upright and balanced as you each bring your lifted (outside) knee across the center and aim to touch each other's lifted knees together in front of you. After you have played around for a while, face the other direction and repeat the pose on the other side.

Step 7: Have each partner come up with a movement or posture you can do together. Be creative and safe; there is no right or wrong here.

Step 8: On a big piece of paper, create a joint expression of the fun, physical time you just shared. You may create independently but together, or allow each person's color and lines to inform what you put on the page.

This exercise of sharing physical and creative space with a trusted loved one nourishes the PM brain and soaks it with oxytocin, the bonding chemical. It is very uplifting to touch and laugh together. Did you notice that your creative resources were close to the surface in this happy, connected environment? Perhaps this carries over in to life: the next time you get stuck on a project, try creating in the same space as someone you feel close to.

Coworking

This principle of "coworking," like parallel play or meditating in a room full of people, soothes our midbrain and amplifies our productivity. Group energy is invigorating and inspiring. We feel like we are a part of something, even when we are doing our own thing. People are more motivated when working in a shared space and, even when completing a different project from everyone else, tend to put more effort and commitment to the task at hand. The simple presence of another being improves and supports us.

The Joy Habit

Another benefit to getting out of the house and connecting to the outer world and people in it is all the joy that awaits us. It's true that there are few places happier than our own homes; however, in the wide, beautiful, magical world outside our doors there lie opportunities and chance meetings we wouldn't have even considered. Furthermore, when we head out while being open to the enriching things that *could* happen, they usually *do*.

Joy, and anticipating joy, are habits of the mind. When the PM brain busies itself avoiding pain and lamenting loneliness, there is little room for joy to enter. If, instead, we acknowledge and actively seek that which inspires and uplifts us, we are nourished on all levels. Commit yourself to seeking and acknowledging joy rather than looking for what's missing. This joy habit reprograms your brain and really changes its size and shape in some areas. That effect is amplified if you apply some meditation or movement along with the quest for joy. The next chapter talks more about cultivating this sustained upliftedness through the neocortex, or neomammalian brain.

Chapter 13
Human

JUST AS YOU HAVE been going through a process of personal evolution through this book, so the human brain has been evolving over generations. As our species learns and grows, those lessons are reflected in the size, shape, structure, and function of the brain. Human brains are the only ones that have a highly developed neocortex—this part of the brain wraps around the hind- and midbrains and is characterized by many folds (sulci)—and prefrontal cortex, which is responsible for personality expression, planning, anticipating outcomes, and other complex cognitive processes. The brain is not the only thing that makes us human.

Humans, along with a handful of other animals, express altruism (seemingly selfless care for one another), shame, and rituals. We have social codes and complex language, including written symbols. Despite our ability to foresee outcomes and plan ahead, we mess things up all the time and have the ability to feel badly about it and learn from it. We go through a similar learning curve with our creative expression: visualize an outcome, go through the process, wind up dissatisfied with the end result. This is where our higher reason can interfere with our creative endeavors. Let the following exercise help you hearken back to your simpler, mammalian habits as you enjoy the present moment and create without shame.

Exercise: Let It Be Awful: Creating for Creation's Sake

You have permission to dream … and make really bad art. Really bad. Like, what were you thinking?! Because those initial pieces of truthful expression are important, no matter how they look. Be playful! Let the process be the key aspect of this, not the outcome.

Step 1: Settle into a reclined relaxation posture. Deepen your breath; allow the surface to hold you as you release layers of tension. Turn up the corners of your mouth and soften your eyeballs behind their closed lids. Notice your personal process of releasing tension; how do you unwind and let go of those areas?

Step 2: Create something you never have before. Use a new medium, style, or subject. Witness the nay-sayer as you might in a mindfulness practice: letting it wash over you without attending it. Focus, instead, on the creative act itself.

Step 3: When you are finished, no matter how it turned out, feel a sense of achievement for having endeavored. The victory was in taking action, not in the outcome.

This is a truth that I hope you can carry through each creation you attempt. Create for creation's sake—for the purpose of doing. Trust yourself and your vision and know that your output is one marker on an entire process of *becoming*.

Connecting with the creative soul is a course we cycle through again and again. An important aspect of that cycle is the poor or not-pretty things that come out of us. Stay playful, experiment, and relax as you just let it be awful.

Change Your Brain, Change Your Life

Like making art in a new way, our attempts at personal change are often clumsy and ugly. We used to be taught that we had a set number of brain cells and when we killed them, that was it—they were gone! We now know that the brain is genuinely plastic and total change is more possible for us. The brain can change shape and size in different areas and build new pathways within itself. Neuroplasticity gives us hope even if something has gone terribly wrong for the brain—there is corrective action we can take in cases of brain injury or stroke. This holds true on smaller levels too, such as rewiring old pains and learning new behaviors.

Research shows that meditation thickens parts of the brain associated with the areas responsible for our ability to reflect upon and offer meaning to the past, project into the future, strategize, and have greater compassion and empathy. As discussed above, these are parts of the brain that set us apart from most other animals.

What we focus on becomes real to us in deeper and more precise ways. What we do not focus on remains unobserved and parts of the brain responsible for noticing it will not develop as much as areas we attend to. In this way, we rehearse our emotional and relational habits and get very adept at feeling and perceiving basically the same way day after day. We have the same routines and beliefs repeating themselves within us on an almost continual basis. We automatically follow the same path in the brain again and again because it is the habit.

Cultivating new emotional habits and transforming underlying beliefs forge new neuronal connections. At first, we have to focus on making the change. When we catch ourselves repeating old habits, thinking in patterned ways, or rehearsing beliefs that no longer serve us, we higher-thinking humans have the choice to consciously redirect. When you identify the person you wish to become, be it happier, more artistic, calmer, etc., and dedicate yourself in small, meaningful ways to practice being that person, your brain will eventually rewire itself to comply with that personal vision and intention.

Being Human

Despite our best intentions and most committed practice, we still slip away from our ideal vision of ourselves. We become mean or worried; we fail at things that are important to us. It is validating to know that even joyful people feel anger, sadness, and fear. Even spiritual people can behave like jerks. Every human is human!

 Exercise: Gaining Inspiration from Dark Emotions

A thriving, creative person views these commonly uncomfortable emotions and lapses in excellence as fuel and inspiration, so even in the darkest places, there is a hint of delight. This exercise gives you a template to live into that truth.

Step 1: Have a bad day. You don't need to make that happen just so you can complete this exercise. Live a normal life—bad days happen. When you catch one, either because of a current situation, hormonal shifts, or trauma resurfacing, come back to this exercise and use that darkness as a creative force.

Step 2: Express the darkness in your own fashion. It may come out as images, melodies, or words. Allow it to flow from you; it may be intense. Do not interfere with its process. Judgment has no place here. The darkness has its own presence and intelligence. Let it out.

Step 3 (optional): Relax or care for yourself in a healthy way, such as deep breathing, a walk, or one of the exercises in this book.

Step 4: Review your work. What does it say to you? What is the unmet need and are you able to cultivate that quality? If there were a moral to its story, what might it be?

Step 5: Create a piece that is a response to your expressed darkness. You may choose the same medium or create with different materials. What do you want to say, convey, or offer to that darker part?

Now that you have expressed, witnessed, and acknowledged a darker or painful aspect, is there a shift within you? Once we externalize held pain, we open closed places. Depending upon your history, this truth may not be evident at first. Whenever you approach gloom, overwhelm, or despair you can repeat this exercise. In time, you will experience a lightening. When that happens, you may bask in openness or consciously fill those places with divine qualities and self-assurance.

Be aware that you do not get caught in a dark, brooding way of being. Although we may be genetically, chemically, or behaviorally predisposed, depression is not our natural state. It's human to feel that way sometimes. Continue applying the principles of this book to channel your painful experiences and emotions into self-expression while remembering that your creative essence is divinely joyful. It's okay when we're human; it's lovely when we're divine.

Human Condition

As humans, we are more alike than different. Your sadness feels the same as the sadness of those in other countries. The way you feel about your children is basically the same as parents who have completely different customs and beliefs. We all get hungry, tired, and sad. When you laugh, it's similar to the uplifting release I feel when I laugh. Most of us enjoy sneezing and abhor hiccups. Humans around the world have similar wants, needs, and emotions.

Our commonality is one of the reasons we travel the world to engage with the art of other humans. Books are translated into many languages. Music moves us to tears. Even in lineages well outside our own culture or from completely different times, art offers powerful reflections of the human condition. Yoga tradition teaches that we are one. Society teaches that we are separate, resources are limited, and we must compete with one another. Such programming keeps us feeling isolated and impoverished.

Human behavior studies reveal that stimuli in our environment, such as words on billboards and song lyrics, even when we are not paying attention to them, affect how we feel and treat one another. Watch or listen to the first sixty seconds of a news report and then read that sentence again. What are the implications? The mainstream world around us seems to be set up to keep us separate and afraid; in other words, living into our base, reptilian nature rather than putting effort toward our uplifted, creative one.

Now that you are awake to this idea, you may sense the world with a different kind of discernment. You are more likely to notice the negative programming that appeals to the inner lizard and keeps us selfish and separate. You will perceive humor that is more mean than witty, political messages more frightening than informative. From this discernment, you will cull your environment, choosing that which feeds and inspires uplifting action and true self-expression. In order to stay connected to the creative essence, we must be in a place of safety, self-connection, and inspiration.

Most folks go through life loving one another ... unless they cut us off in traffic or say something unkind behind our backs. Then all bets are off. We are creative, peaceful, and compassionate until we aren't. With established spiritual practice and some creative thinking, we are able to perceive that maybe we got cut off because we were driving slowly in the fast lane, or that person had a family emergency we don't know about, or their own egoism makes them drive like a maniac. What that person gossiped about us had a grain of truth—we can work on those things in ourselves. They spoke unkindly because they think unkindly—of *themselves*, that is. Projection is a thing. The next exercise lets you work on it a bit.

 ### Exercise: Why Is That Guy Such a Jerk?!: Understanding Your Triggers

Carl Jung taught us about our "shadows." Not the dark patch on the ground that walks with us on sunny days; this kind of shadow is the psychological dumping ground of all human aspects we don't like to see within ourselves. This exercise helps you identify your shadow so you are less likely to see it—and hate it—in others. The more we accept all aspects of ourselves, the more compassion we can offer to others who are also living out their humanness.

Step 1: Who really bugs you? It may be a sibling, coworker, or person at the car dealership's service desk.

Step 2: What bugs you about that person? Write down as many traits as you can think of. If no one person bugs you, you can just make a general list of things you don't like about other people.

Step 3: Get really, really curious. In what ways do you possess each of those attributes you listed? Even though you don't like to admit it—you have worked hard to distance yourself from those traits—notice how you actually have them in some way... Hey, man, don't project your resistance on to me. I am not the one who discovered this universal truth. Stay curious and you will perceive how it is so.

To answer the question in the title of this exercise, that guy is a jerk because we are all jerks. It's human nature. As creative souls, we have the ability to transcend that human nature. You are equipped to perceive alternative reasons and realities *and* you have the internal resources to use others' hurtful behavior to fuel your inspiration. In this way, you transmute their poison into medicine and move in the direction of unitive consciousness. I once heard the Dalai Lama speak of burning others' *karma* for them, through our own compassion and nonattachment. That is a deep form of service to humanity and requires great purity and connection to one's true Self. The following exercise gives you tools to stay connected to your essential Self, even in times of interpersonal strife.

 Exercise: Burning *Karma* through Neutral Awareness or the Virtue of Joy

Before embarking upon the steps of this exercise, let's do a quick *karma* refresher. Earlier in this book we spoke of *karma* as a path of service and effort, guided by personal purpose, or *dharma*. *Karma* indicates the action and its fruit, or outcome. Despite pop culture's quest for "good *karma*," we are truly seeking no *karma* and wish to burn off the *karma* we have already accrued. You can check out some of the yoga books in this book's recommended reading list for more information about this concept.

Step 1: Be *karma*-free. Just kidding—many cultures believe that as long as you have a body it is proof that you are not free from the residue of your previous actions. However, if you can accept circumstances and the people involved as they come, you are on a strong path to freedom. Do your best to perceive all people and situations as neutral, noting it is only our projections of right, wrong, and wanting that give them a charge. As you hold this state of equanimity, you limit the amount of *karma* incurred.

Step 2: Enter a situation you find happy or exciting. Do your best to maintain this accepting, compassionate, neutral perspective. Using the mindful awareness approach from previous chapters, witness the ways in which you lose equanimity. What triggers your excitement? Can you discern the difference between the limited emotion of happiness and the pervasive virtue of joy? In this step, you may allow a sense of joy to flow through you, noticing that it does not impact neutrality. Joy is a virtue, like compassion, benevolence, and generosity. Like each divine quality, there is joy available in all things.

Joy In All Things

When we are being our true selves, living in alignment with a vision of what is best and real for us, answering to our own authority rather than programming and "shoulds," a sense of joy arises. Joy is qualitatively different from happiness. There is a come-down from happiness, a perception of lack once it is gone. We may feel sad that we are no longer happy. Joy, on the other hand, is available to us in even the darkest of moments. The following exercise can help get you in touch with that.

 Exercise: Getting In Touch with Joy

This exercise guides you through a process of moving through emotions to discover joy. This process takes you beyond your verbal processing and asks you to trust yourself. Let your memories, body, and imagination guide you.

Step 1: Consider a time when you have felt deeply despairing, alone, or hopeless. You may be moving through such a difficulty in your life even now. Let your eyes close as you set your body in comfort and put yourself back to that time. You may imagine yourself in it, as if it were happening now, or watch it like a movie.

Step 2: Observe the physical feelings that occur alongside this grief. Where does it live in your body? How does it make you breathe? What happens to the quality and content of the thoughts moving through your mind during that dark time?

Step 3: Select a song that consistently makes you cry. Alternatively, you may select a song that accompanies the phase you are remembering. Let the song be appropriately despairing and play it as you select five colors of crayon, pencil, pastel, or paint. Do not overthink the color selection.

Step 4: Continuing to play the sad song on repeat and holding your connection to the memory of hopelessness, use your nondominant hand to express the emotions. Let your body be a conduit for feelings, so that each stroke or swipe at the page is an emotional representation. Be truthful in this action by not *thinking* about how to express. Your body already knows how to say what is. Get out of its way. If you start to think, tune in to the song instead, allowing all of your wandering thoughts to merge with the music. Your nondominant hand fills the page with shape and color, not for the sake of art or beauty, but for truth.

Step 5: When you feel done, or have expressed what your body wished to, put the page facedown or cover the canvas and spend five to ten minutes on a relaxation or structured movement sequence from one of the previous chapters. Upon its completion, sit tall and close your eyes, basking in the sense of vitality or relaxation.

Step 6: Without looking at your piece, hold that invigorated or relaxed sense and select one to three more colors. Breathing deeply, gaze upon these colors and imbue them with a sense of upliftedness, well-being, kindness, and healing. Using your nondominant hand again, reveal your previous work and let the colors interact with what you laid down earlier. Imagine these new colors are offering exactly what you needed in that moment of despair.

In real life, we can remember the process of this exercise. On some level of perception, even in the darkest times, joy is available to us. The next time life shocks you with something painful, seek a connection to the virtue of joy. From where are those soothing "colors" available to you?

The human brain and its associated psychological habits offer a path to creative awareness and enlightenment. Inspiration from who we truly are—and our capacity to move toward that true Self—keep us open to new perceptions. We can combine habits and truth to create something never seen or heard before. Our perceptual shifts and intentions toward the creative Self change not only what we believe about ourselves but also how we interact with the outer world. The following chapter builds on this shift, offering a broader view of your creative potential.

Chapter 14
Being

WHAT IS CREATIVITY AND why do we create? When people learn to meditate, meditation itself is not the end goal. We meditate to access a peace and stillness within ourselves or acquire spiritual wisdom. Similarly, our stories and pictures are not the end-all, be-all in our creative endeavors. *Life itself* is our ultimate creative act.

When we consciously create our existence, we are in a state of true Being. Being, as opposed to doing, involves accepting who we are, what we are made of, and the habits, beliefs, desires, and gifts that shape us. In this chapter, you will live into your Being-ness by exploring what it means to be you and experimenting with your potential to create a joyful, authentic life.

Transcendent Humanity

There comes a time when we have gained enough insight into ourselves that we are fully ready to claim our truth and live in the world we wish to create. As discussed previously, many animals are able to plan and make choices. They form families and communities (or I could say pods, gaggles, herds, schools, murders, prides, etc.), they war amongst factions, and they have death rituals. Do they hope and pray? Maybe. Do they meditate and explore transcendent realms? Do they contemplate meaning and purpose? I am not certain. I know that humans do, though.

We have arrived at a phase in our human evolution where our Being-ness can move beyond the neomammalian perspective and enjoy an entirely new phase of consciousness. What was reserved throughout our history for sages, physicists, ministers, and mystics is accessible to all of us. Much of the world's esoteric wisdom, previously reserved for students who earned access over years of humble study, is public knowledge. Granted, it is being taught by flawed humans or disseminated out of context; however, your own direct experience with spiritual practice provides you with insights about the deeper meaning, beyond the words of the teachings.

The secret wisdom of the ages has been unleashed upon the public alongside the public's readiness to do personal reflection and daily practice in order to access the meaning and purpose behind the words. The following exercise supports you in cultivating your own path to a direct experience of divine wisdom.

 Exercise: Daily Practice

"Daily practice," what the yogis call *sadhana,* is a well-studied phenomenon. Whether you are an athlete, musician, spiritualist, writer, painter, mathematician, or engineer, daily practice is key to refining and developing your skills. If we miss even one day, our prowess begins to slip. For those of us on a path of personal evolution, which requires great commitment due to mainstream society's predispositions (discussed later this chapter), daily practice is a key component of our evolution. The following system will support you in connecting with personal victories and insights.

Step 1: Select a personally meaningful intention or goal. This can be to increase the speed and accuracy of your musical scales, establish a clearer relationship with heavenly energies, or free yourself from loneliness. Any intention that is important to you is perfect—no need to judge or overthink. The only thing to be cautious of is ensuring that it is *your* intention and does not rely on anyone else.

Step 2: Identify one specific action you can take each day to move in the direction of your intention. Following the examples above, we might say "Run each scale once per day" or "Practice the most difficult scale three times in a row, perfectly, four times per week." "Meditate for twelve minutes every day" or "Identify a divine presence in an everyday moment, every single day." "Three times per week, visit one of my friends/family members and listen without interrupting, then share something personal about myself in return" or "Notice a moment of genuine connection every single day." Note that you may refine this action over time to find what works best for you. As you move in the direction of your intention, the required action may naturally shift.

Step 3: Record the progress of this intention. Be clear about the experiences you have. Note the insights that arise. Remain inspired!

Step 4: The time will come when you feel a sense of mastery over or completion of this goal/intention. Then it is time to move on to another. You may retain the behaviors that led to your uplifted, victorious awareness because they are habits now.

You may continue moving in the direction of your evolution by cultivating a healthy daily practice, one after another. Once an intention becomes established behavior, develop another. Continually following a daily practice inevitably supports us in realizing the true inner creator. In this way, life itself is an act of creation.

YOU'RE the Creator!

Self-mastery is evident when we create the life of our dreams. You came to this world with all you already need to be the perfect version of yourself, living exactly as you wish to. Our skills, aptitudes, and interests are all clues about the person we are meant to be. You possess a unique combination of gifts that only you can offer to the world. When each of us lives in full alignment with those gifts, the world will be a transformed home for us all.

Creativity, for some, is about artistic expression. That has been the focus of most of this book. However, our inventiveness and collective idea-making are other forms of creation. Whatever global/political/ personal issue keeps you up at night already has a solution. For it to be brought into being, however, we cannot be trapped in the corporate machine. It takes courage to step out of societal norms and spend more time freeing our minds and our inner joy. However, that is exactly what needs to happen if the world is going to change. This simple shift in consciousness—each of us connecting to and expressing from our creative soul—is the path to freedom for all humans.

How is very simple. The main point was taught to most of us as children: "Do unto others as you would have them do unto you" or "Love one another." Where the simple message gets lost is in our own egos. We must remember that we are from divine Creation, therefore divine creators. Creative intelligence holds solutions to any problem we experience or can think up. It may not be drawn into reality yet; however, by connecting to your own creative essence you become part of the solution and a creative inspiration for those around you. Explore this in the next exercise.

Exercise: Applying Your Gifts

Get in touch with what makes you special and how you can harness your aptitudes to create the life of your dreams, including a more peaceful, connected world.

Step 1: List the things you or others appreciate about you. Consider talents, personality traits, offerings, etc. This step is easier if you take the question to five people you trust, as well. "I'm reading this book and it wants me to ask you what you appreciate about me…"

Step 2: In what ways do you contribute to making the world better in action? Consider within your household (recycling, buying items used rather than new, teaching your children the value of "service," etc.), community (picking up litter, making food for an ailing neighbor, supporting local farmers, etc.), and globally (petitioning against and refusing to purchase products from multinational corporations, sponsoring a child in an underprivileged nation, volunteering time to missions, etc.).

Step 3: In what ways do you make the world better from your own upliftedness? Consider the impact your peace of mind has within your household/job, community, and even globally. If we are in some way a unified consciousness, as yoga teachings and other great thinkers/scientists suggest, then your upliftedness is valuable to all.

When we acknowledge the connectedness between all humans and live as if our actions are of value, not only to ourselves but others, we create a more conscientious and uplifted world. You create not only on the smaller scale of self-expression, but on the grand human scale as well through your everyday thoughts and actions.

From the perspective of unified consciousness, you may consider that each thought you have is like a ripple in the collective thought-field, or a prayer for the outcome associated with the thought. For the last ten years or so, much has been said about the idea that our thoughts create our reality. Consider that every thought you think, whether conscious or automatic, is a prayer. Our random thoughts may be requests for the divine. We create with each belief, image, and speculation. As a creative person, you can harness this power and apply the power of your mind to the good of all humanity. The next exercise takes that idea one step further.

 Exercise: Thoughts Create Reality

In your personal growth journey, you have likely encountered the idea that our thoughts create our reality. This often speaks to our ongoing perceptions and the way we filter and give meaning to events. There is also the idea that our thoughts are magnetic, drawing our expectations, fears, and hopes into being. What reality do you wish to create?

Step 1: Take fifteen seconds and list some of the problems you see in the world. Do not spend more than fifteen seconds—there are many and you might fall into despair before you even make it to step 2. Trust that the first few that come out of you are the ones that relate best to your individual gifts, aptitudes, and passions.

Step 2: You made it here! Now, become aware of your thoughts as they pass through your mind on an average day. There are lots of them; it's okay if you forget to witness sometimes. Simply notice, whenever you think of it (or set a timer), "What am I thinking right now?"

Step 3: Follow that awareness up with some intentionality: "If these thoughts were true, what kind of world would that be?

Is that the world I wish to create?" If yes, excellent. If no, continue to the next step.

Step 4: Now that you are conscious of your thoughts and your power as a creator, imagine something wonderful for the world. Relate this conscious creative thought to an item on your list from step 1. If you think this thought and combine it with feelings of thankfulness, joy, and hope, you are engaged in a very powerful practice.

Step 5 (optional): What happens for some people in this exercise is that they begin to dream of or have spontaneous ideas about concrete actions that they could take to align with the thoughts of step 4. Remember, every thought we have is a prayer for its material existence. If we are contemplating the end of some kind of strife, we will inevitably receive ideas about how we can end it. This is a process of divine cocreation.

Inspiration engages us in creating a new reality, the same way it impels us to create art. This is not about cultivating a "God Complex"; rather, growing a faithful relationship with ourselves as creative beings. We are of Creation; therefore, we are creative. Divine creative forces wish to support our creative powers in small and large ways. When we feel hopeless or concerned about the state of the world, it is simply a cue to direct our creative resources.

If we are the creators of our own lives then there must be some kind of signpost or way of marking the path so that we know we are heading in the right direction. Since we are cocreating with life (or God, divine forces, quanta, our future Selves, or however you conceptualize it), we can keep an eye out for feedback as we choose our thoughts and live into being the creator.

Exercise: Accessing Divine Guidance

Since you are cocreating with divine Creation, you may trust that force to offer you continual guidance. Here are steps to take in order to prove this to yourself. Stay open to how messages and hints appear, and, of course, be creative and inspired in how you interpret them.

Step 1: As with previous exercises, be intentional about your thoughts, words, and actions as you move toward the life of your dreams. Request guidance or feedback about these intentions and actions.

Step 2: Assume that the answer to your request is forthcoming. Keep all five senses open and engaged. Note coincidences, including what song comes on the radio, words that jump out at you, wafts of inexplicable aromas, or overheard snippets of conversation.

Step 3: Sometimes these signposts will suggest the cultivation of a virtue. They may also give clues to your next step. Sometimes they request a minor adjustment or recalibration.

Step 4: Be thankful for whatever messages you receive, no matter how subtly or strangely they come. Believe in this kind of subtle support and follow the "recommendations" that seem to be coming through.

Connecting to the creative soul and fashioning the life you ideally wish to live is a joint process. None of us does this alone. You are a cocreator with your creative soul, and with the divine essence of life. Connecting to other humans who are living into their own Being-ness is another way of cultivating creative connection.

Creative Community

As discussed in previous chapters, we are healthier when surrounded by like-minded others who see and respect us. As creative beings, it is beneficial to create life with others who share our vision and missions. This can mean joining groups who are acting on behalf of causes we believe in or becoming a member of a knitting, singing, or painting group. What is important is the supportive, collaborative energy.

Share your work with others. Let them know the thoughts you are consciously cultivating and show them your personal creative endeavors. You can develop your craft by requesting pieces of feedback, be it complimentary or constructive. (I recommend the former when you are getting started and the latter before you go public.) Speaking of going public, *show your work*. Do readings, hang your efforts in local cafes, perform in recitals. The more we put ourselves out there as creative beings, the more we inspire others to pursue their own creative gifts. The world is ready for this level of healing. If you are afraid or insecure, try the next exercise.

Exercise: Put It Out There: Showing Your Stuff/Self

Many of us are comfortable creating in private. Through exercises like those in this book, we may even move beyond self-judgment and fear of what comes out of us. Showing it to someone else is another scary step to take. Showing it to the world … that might be too far. But it isn't!

Step 1: Select ten pieces that mean something to you. These will likely be associated with deep emotional release or externalizing something you held in for a long, long time. They probably reflect something profoundly true for you … and you may not know exactly what that is.

Step 2: Of those ten pieces, select five that you think might be "good" by conventional (and I use that word loosely) standards. What is unique? What truly speaks to you? Which has received praise from others?

Step 3: Show your stuff. You can be creative with this as well. If your pieces are dances, go to a park or dance club and move through them. If it is written work, speak them publicly at an open mic night, poetry slam, or "speakers' corner." If it is visual art, find somewhere to show it or hang copies on bulletin boards. It may seem strange to share in informal or subversive ways; however, these are steps in revealing yourself.

Throughout the course of this book you have learned to connect to and create with your creative essence. Now share your gifts, insights, and inspiration!

Conclusion

As you have moved through the process of this book, you have faced many of your demons, released and transmuted old pain, and connected to a deeper sense of worth and inner knowing. By revealing more of these parts of yourself to the world at large, you impel others to do the same. The more each of us connects with our creative essence, the more freedom and joy we are capable of. Another way to say that is, by sharing your creative truth, you connect others to the truth within them. As each of us aligns with our creative essence, we are less likely to carry misery and spread it around the world.

By becoming more creative, compassionate beings, we come up with more ideas to change the current global status quo. We are less tolerant of dehumanizing groups based on socioeconomics, politics, or geographic locations. Unity begets unity. In this way, you are experiencing yoga and creativity as personal and global activism. You don't have to become a banner-waving activist; the creative process you took through this book is enough. Now share it with others. Your authentic voice is important. We are listening.

Once we have learned about the obstacles in our own way, explored five paths for connecting beyond those blocks, and accepted our neurological heritage as embodied spirits, we can set to the task of living this life. *Yoga for the Creative Soul* is a book you can return to again and again through the rest of your life and—although your personal growth themes and *karma* will be similar—you will be different every time you come back. Throughout the book, I discussed underlying yoga therapy principles. Yoga therapy supports you in understanding your mind—the emotions, beliefs, perceptions, and choices that lead us to joy or despair. We are transformed by choosing our own perspectives and taking conscious, intentional action. Stay connected to your deep motivation. Follow these exercises and practices and get into a creative flow, then keep it up!

Thank you for sharing the journey and engaging with this book. I wish you much joy, freedom, and insight on this yogic path of connecting with your creative soul.

Glossary

Abhinivesa: Fear of death/change

Ahimsa: Nonviolence

Ajna chakra: "Command" *chakra* at forehead

Anahata chakra: "Unstruck" *chakra* at heart

Ananda: Bliss

Anandamaya kosha: The innermost sheath, bliss, spirit

Apanasana: Ball Pose

Aparigraha: Nonattachment

Ardha chandrasana: Half Moon Pose

Asana: Physical posture or pose in yoga

Asmita: Egoism

Asteya: Non-stealing

Avidya: Spiritual ignorance

Balasana: Child's Pose

Bhagavad Gita: Foundational spiritual text of yoga

Bhakti: Path of emotion, love, devotion

Bhakta: One who follows the *Bhakti* Path

Bhujangasana: Cobra Pose

Brahmacharya: Moderation, continence, retaining and directing sexual energy to the highest

Chakras: Energy centers, "wheels"

Deviasana: Goddess Pose

Dhanurasana: Bow Pose

Dharana: Concentration

Dharma: Duty, purpose

Dhyana: Meditative state

Dvesha: Aversion

Ishvara pranidhana: Surrender

Jnana: Knowledge

Jnani: One who follows the *Jnana* Path

Karma: Action brings reaction; outcome

Karma Yoga: Path of yoga by which self-realization occurs through work/selfless service

Kati chakrasana: Standing Twisted Posture

Kosha: Sheath or layer

Klesa: Obstacle, hindrance to enlightenment

Kumbhaka: Breath retention

Kundalini Upanishad: Ancient scripture outlining bioenergy techniques

Makarasana: Crocodile Pose

Manas: Mind/emotion

Manipura chakra: "Hidden gem" at solar plexus

Maya: Illusory, material reality

Nadi: Energy channel

Niyama: Observance

Prana: Bioenergy or life force

Pranayama: Breath control/direction/prolongation

Pratyahara: Sensory mastery

Puraka: Prolonged inhale

Raga: Attachment

Raja: The "Royal" path; from the *Yoga Sutras*,
     psychology, meditation

Rajas: Active, lustful, hyper, greedy

Rechaka: Prolonged exhale

Sadhana: Remembrance, daily practice

Samadhi: Union, enlightenment

Samkalpa: Intention

Samskara: Grooves, patterns, pathways

Samtosha: Contentment

Satya: Truthfulness

Savasana: Corpse Pose

Shalabhasana: Locust Pose

Simhasana: Lion Pose

Sunyaka: Breath suspension

Svadhyaya: Study of self or scripture

Talasana: Palm Tree Pose

Tamasic: Inactive, dull, depressed, low vitality

Tantra: "To expand and liberate," path of energetic awareness and connection

Tapas: Discipline, effort, routine, austerity

Taittiriya Upanishad: Ancient scripture outlining the layers of being, from food to joy

Uttanasana: Standing Forward Bend

Vijnana: Discerning intellect

Virabhadrasana I: Warrior I Pose

Virabhadrasana II: Warrior II Pose

Yama: Restraint

Yastikasana: Stick Pose

Recommended Resources

THIS SECTION OFFERS YOU means of continuing this journey through yoga, creativity, and personal healing/growth. First, what to do when your brain/heart/soul breaks open—it's not always pretty. Next, prudent things to consider when finding an art/yoga class, yoga therapist, psychotherapist/counselor, or body worker. Finally, a list of recommended reading will follow. May you receive all that you require on this journey.

Getting Help: Reach Out

If memories, bodily reactions, stirred-up emotions, or any uncomfortable experience starts to feel like too much, it's okay to reach out for help right away. I used to not call crisis lines because I didn't want to waste their time. As a former crisis line worker, let me assure you that no issue is too small to reach out about. If you are genuinely experiencing something you need support with: *reach out.*

If your call isn't appropriate for the line you called, the person at the other end will make sure of at least two things before they end the call. First, they will ensure you have the correct numbers to call. Second, they will make sure you are safe to wrap up and end the current call.

You can find local crisis line numbers through a simple web search: your town, province/state, and the phrase "twenty-four–hour crisis line." For example, "Springfield Kentucky 24 hour crisis line" will give you a list of options if you live near there. You can even search internationally, as some countries have 1-800 numbers staffed continually for a variety of specific issues.

The first few pages of the telephone book typically list local crisis lines. Some of them may be specific to issues that you do not identify as your own. Call them anyway and they will be able to support you or point you to someone who can. I do not recommend calling 911 unless you are in imminent mortal danger.

While crisis line calls may be time-limited and not offer the resources to go deeply, they are highly beneficial in helping you remain safe and connected. Under the best of circumstances, they reconnect you to your inner resources, where your answers and well-being are continually vital.

Finding a Yoga Therapist

There are many schools of yoga and approaches to this vast tradition. That diversity is evident in the realm of yoga therapy as well. Some questions you may wish to ask a potential yoga therapist are:

- Where did you receive your training as a yoga therapist?

- Is your education accredited or are you registered with an association like the International Association of Yoga Therapists?

- Do you follow a prescriptive approach to physical/mental conditions or will I be looked at comprehensively?

- Do you work outside-in (from symptoms) or inside-out (from state of mind)?

- How adaptable are the postures and breathing exercises you teach?

- What is the role of yoga philosophy in your sessions?

- Will we discuss lifestyle?

You may also share a short, simple intention with potential yoga therapists to hear how their approach may align with your personal vision. The following sections offer you more salient questions.

Finding a Yoga/Art Class That's Right for You

The ongoing education, practice, and community associated with taking classes is invaluable in supporting our growth and daily practice. Here are some factors to consider:

- What education/experience/professional affiliations/ certification does the teacher have?

- What is the teacher's educational philosophy?

- Do you click?

- Can I respect and follow direction from this person?

- How much does it cost?

- What are the short- and long-term costs of *not* pursuing this?

Finding a Psychotherapist, Body Worker, or Other Professional Support

Similar to the inspiration, motivation, and help offered by classes, one-on-one healing experiences are key to our development and well-being. In a healthy life, it is wise to procure a personal wellness team. In addition to the questions considered when finding a class, ask the following:

- Based on evidence, is this safe?

- Do I feel safe?

(Those two questions are asking very different things. For example, although physician support is safe based on evidence, individual physicians may not be trustworthy. This is true for all professions.)

- Is any of this covered by health insurance/work benefits?

- What makes me believe this is the best intervention for me at this time?

- Where relevant, is this person respectful in when/how they touch my body?

- Where relevant, is the quality of physical contact what I am looking for/need?

- Am I comfortable offering feedback to this person?

As you continue building a team on your own behalf, you will come to discover other questions that are also relevant and meaningful to you. Be sure to add those to the list, too.

Recommended Reading

THERE ARE MORE GREAT books out there than I can possibly name. Below is a list of a few that appeal to diverse personalities and create powerful impacts. Many of them have their own recommended reading lists in the back. Enjoy the discovery process and remember you don't have to read every page of every book. Receive what is useful and carry on.

Andrews, Ted. *Animal Speak.* Woodbury, MN: Llewellyn Publications, 1993.

Brand, Russell. *Revolution.* New York: Random House, 2014.

Butera, Kristen, and Staffan Elgelid. *Yoga Therapy: A Personalized Approach for Your Active Lifestyle.* New York: Human Kinetics, 2017.

Butera, Robert. *Meditation for Your Life.* Woodbury, MN: Llewellyn Publications, 2011.

_____. *The Pure Heart of Yoga.* Woodbury, MN: Llewellyn Publications, 2009.

Butera, Robert, and Erin Byron. *Llewellyn's Complete Book of Mindful Living.* Woodbury, MN: Llewellyn Publications, 2016.

Butera, Robert, Staffan Elgelid, and Erin Byron. *Yoga Therapy for Stress and Anxiety.* Woodbury, MN: Llewellyn Publications, 2015.

Cameron, Julia. *Artist's Way: A Spiritual Path to Higher Creativity.* New York: Penguin Putnam, 1992.

Canfield, Jack. *The Success Principles, 10th Anniversary Edition.* New York: HarperCollins, 2015.

Diggins, Gary. *Tuning the Eardrums: Listening as a Mindful Practice.* Victoria, Canada: Friesen Press, 2016.

Dillard, Sherrie. *Sacred Signs & Symbols: Awaken to the Messages and Synchronicities that Surround You.* Woodbury, MN: Llewellyn Publications, 2017.

Easwaran, Ecknath. *The Bhagavad Gita.* Tomales, California: Nilgiri Press, 2007.

_____. *The Upanishads.* Tomales, California: Nilgiri Press, 2007.

Edwards, Betty. *Drawing on the Right Side of the Brain.* New York: Penguin Putnam, 1999.

Gawain, Shakti. *Creative Visualization, Anniversary Edition.* Toronto, Canada: New World Publishing, 2016.

Gilbert, Elizabeth. *Big Magic: Creative Living Beyond Fear.* New York: Penguin Random House, 2015.

Neff, Kristin. *Self-Compassion.* London, UK: Hodder and Stoughton, 2011.

Pressfield, Steven, and Shawn Coyne. *The War of Art.* New York: Black Irish Entertainment, 2002.

Satchidananda, Sri Swami (trans.). *The Yoga Sutras of Patanjali.* Yogaville, VA: Integral Yoga Publications, 1978.

Taylor, Matthew J. (ed.). *Fostering Creativity in Rehabilitation.* New York: Nova Science Publishers, 2015.

Tharp, Twyla. *The Creative Habit.* New York: Simon & Schuster, 2003.

Van Der Kolk, Bessel. *The Body Keeps the Score.* New York: Viking Press, 2014.

Wunthow, Robert. *Creative Spirituality: The Way of the Artist.* London, UK: University of California Press, 2001.